POST-INDUSTRIAL SOCIALISM

Post-Industrial Socialism critically analyses recent developments in Leftist political thought. It charts new directions in the economy and the effects they have had on traditional models of social welfare and orthodox approaches to social policy.

The book begins with an outline of post-industrial socialism by differentiating it from other trends in contemporary theory. Adrian Little builds upon a blend of traditional socialist concepts, such as universalism, solidarity and social justice, and incorporates elements of ecological, anti-racist and feminist politics. He presents a form of citizenship in which individuals and the state have economic rights and obligations, as well as civil, political and social rights.

In demonstrating the limitations of the welfare state and the associated concept of citizenship, this book suggests that we need to renew socialist welfare theory through the evaluation of universal welfare provision and a policy of breaking the link between work and income.

Adrian Little is Senior Lecturer in Politics at Nene College of Higher Education, Northampton.

POST-INDUSTRIAL SOCIALISM

Towards a new politics of welfare

Adrian Little

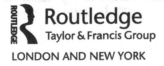

Routledge
Taylor & Francis Group

LONDON AND NEW YORK

First published 1998
by Routledge
2 Park Square, Milton Park, Abingdon, Oxon, OX14 4RN

Simultaneously published in the USA and Canada
by Routledge
605 Third Avenue, New York, NY 10017

*Routledge is an imprint of the Taylor & Francis Group,
an informa business*

Typeset in Baskerville by
M Rules

British Library Cataloguing in Publication Data
A catalogue record for this book is available from the British Library

Library of Congress Cataloguing in Publication Data
A catalogue record for this book has been requested

ISBN 13: 978-0-415-17194-6 (pbk)
ISBN 13: 978-0-415-17193-9 (hbk)

Publisher's Note
The publisher has gone to great lengths to ensure the quality of this
reprint but points out that some imperfections in the original
may be apparent

TO SINEAD

CONTENTS

ACKNOWLEDGEMENTS

The inspiration for this book was my encounter with the radical theoretical debates on welfare in Europe in the course of writing my earlier book *The Political Thought of André Gorz*. It seemed remarkable that these radical ideas were not finding any real currency in the realms of political and social theory and social policy in the United Kingdom. Hopefully the argument constructed in this book will demonstrate the relevance of these theoretical debates to our understanding of socialism and the new directions in policy-making which are currently emerging.

Patrick Proctor has supported this project wholeheartedly, as have the rest of the people involved in the production of the book at Routledge. Two anonymous readers provided detailed critical comments that alerted me to a range of pertinent issues which I had to address. I am grateful to my colleagues in the School of Social Studies at Nene College for their comments on earlier drafts and papers on which much of this book is based. I have benefited enormously from discussions with Wolfgang Deicke, Gordon Hughes, Andrew Pilkington, Keith Sharp and Chris Winch. Gordon Hughes, in particular, must be thanked for his assiduous reading of each chapter and his help in collaborative research. I should also acknowledge the help of a variety of people who helped me formulate my ideas when the book was in an embryonic stage, such as Andrew Dobson, Robert Eccleshall, Vincent Geoghegan, André Gorz, John Keane, Michael Kenny and Conrad Lodziak. I have enjoyed agreeing and disagreeing with all of the above at various times. Ultimately, though, the responsibility for any errors or inaccuracies lies in my hands.

INTRODUCTION
The context of post-industrial socialism

At the beginning of the 1990s Jurgen Habermas posed the question 'What Does Socialism Mean Today?' (Habermas 1990: 3). The answers to such a question will be just as varied now as those perspectives which Habermas originally identified. Despite the fact that in the late 1990s there has been a rebirth of socialist parties in government in Europe, a synthesised socialist approach to the problems of the current era is not apparent. Certainly, orthodox Marxist, neo-Keynesian and social democratic perspectives remain influential but there is increased evidence that some on the centre Left, such as in the Labour Party in the United Kingdom, are trying to formulate socio-economic programmes around liberalised market mechanisms. Simultaneously, other elements within the socialist canon have sought inspiration through an engagement with the ideas of political ecology. However, none of these approaches has been successful in articulating a unifying socialist ethos which could provide answers to the questions which are thrown up by the global economy or a robust defence against the hegemony of market liberalism. To this extent there has been an ongoing debate over whether it is even relevant to talk of socialism any more (Van Parijs 1995: 3; Kallscheuer 1994). In response to these ideas this book is concerned with outlining the framework of a relatively new Leftist approach to the current era which, following Gorz, is best described as post-industrial socialism. This is not a fully fledged perspective but one which is gathering momentum as advanced capitalism throws up increasingly perplexing questions for which it appears to have no answer. Along with the ideas of Gorz, the growth of the post-industrial Left is reflected in the work of social theorists such as Conrad Lodziak, preceded by Herbert Marcuse, as well as commentators including Claus Offe, Philippe Van Parijs, Bill Jordan and other advocates of guaranteed income schemes which are based upon the need to break the link between income and work.

1

The project of post-industrial socialism

With the exception of the 'liberalised markets' approach mentioned above, there does appear to be one general theme around which these elements of the Left can still unite, the idea that 'the economic system is not a holy of holies but a testing ground' and that a key to socialist strategy should be an attempt 'to find out how much strain the economic system can be made to take in directions that might benefit social needs' (Habermas 1990: 18). The impetus behind the operationalisation of this concept of redrawing the boundaries of economic rationality (Gorz 1989a) lies in a Leftist engagement with radical democracy and normative values. For Habermas, the engagement with the discourses of radical democracy can be used as a mechanism which engenders greater solidarity. In other words, a limitation of economic rationality will not in itself fashion a socialised economy in a deterministic manner but it could be part of a process in which democratic dialogue over the extent of economic mechanisms could lead to a restraint in their operation. Simultaneously, the social process of defining boundaries for market operations entails opening up new spheres for co-operative action in civil society (Keane 1988) or the lifeworld which, in itself, has been imbued with solidaristic values (Habermas 1990). However, this kind of project entails appropriate spaces and opportunities being created in which dialogue can take place, and in turn this requires the reversal of central mechanisms of advanced capitalist reproduction. In this context Anderson notes the importance of two potentially compatible developments – a reduction in working hours and the provision of some form of guaranteed income (Anderson 1994: 19).

These two strategies will be examined in detail later in the book but suffice it to say for the time being that they are central to the understanding of what a 'post-industrial' socialism might actually entail. Put simply, post-industrialism means a break with some of the main features of capitalist industrialism. The notion of reduced working hours *for all* is a key characteristic of post-industrial socialism because it would involve the negation of the ideology of work which substantiates the reproduction of advanced capitalist societies, rather than the reinforcement of industrialist logic which takes place in the new economy. In other words, it undermines the notion that everyone should work or be available for work in any given period. Building upon this premise, some form of guaranteed income would provide a buttress which would enable people to work less and simultaneously acquire greater control over their time usage. Taken alone, either of these measures might be appropriated to reproduce further the capitalist system but taken together they provide a post-industrial dimension which could enhance the regeneration of socialism because it encompasses the limitation of capitalism (although the retention of capital) and the rejection of market-based society (but not necessarily markets).

> Abandoning the reference to socialism would lead also to abandoning any reference to a desirable 'beyond' of capitalism, would lead us to accept this latter as 'natural' and unchangeable, and to speak with a naive idealism of democracy and justice while treating as a negligible quantity the economico-material matrix of capital which, because it demands profitability above all, cannot help but be a source of domination, alienation and violence.
>
> (Gorz 1994: ix)

Gorz, the most well-known post-industrial socialist theorist, is at pains to suggest that we take the most favourable and rational features of the advanced capitalist system and adapt them towards the goals of socialism. His aim is not to create a new socialist *system* (Kallscheuer 1994: 118–19) but to formulate a mode of social organisation in which non-systemic activities and goals are regarded as highly as those which take place in markets or within the ordination of the state. Again there is a post-industrial dimension to this proposition insofar as it centres upon the subversion of systemic objectives such as ever higher profits regardless of distribution, and economic growth regardless of the harmful environmental effects that continued accumulation and consumption brings. To this extent the Left

> consists in viewing the savings of working time as a liberation of time, by virtue of which social individuals should be able to emancipate themselves from the constraints of economic rationality embodied in capital (i.e. in the domination of dead over living labour). To emancipate themselves not by abolishing capital and the sphere of economically rational commodity activities ... but by assigning them a limited and subaltern function in the development of society. In other words the societal objective of productivity gains must be to bring about a contraction of the sphere governed by economic calculation and an expansion of the self-determined, self-organized spheres of activity in which human faculties can develop freely.
>
> (Gorz 1994: 20)

Clearly, these ideas are formulated in opposition to the dominant rationality which governs advanced capitalist societies, and yet, at the same time, they are based on our ability to subject changes which are already taking place in socio-economic circumstances to socialised, non-economic objectives. This provides a different dimension to socialist thought not least because it highlights a firmly Leftist perspective on the new economy which is not the case with other views, such as the stakeholder economy (Hutton 1996), which are firmly grounded in the maintenance of market mechanisms and hierarchy and economic rationality. At the same time the roots of the post-industrial perspective are grounded in contemporary socio-economic changes. Obviously, though, there are considerable barriers to such a programme of social change, the most salient of which involve scepticism about the ability of the state to control market mechanisms so rigorously, especially in the face of ubiquitous globalisation.

Globalisation and the nation state

The growth of a globalised economy is a widely accepted phenomenon which characterises advanced capitalism, although whether this entails a wholly new economic system is clearly open to question (Hirst and Thompson 1996: 47). The globalisation thesis would have us believe that nation states are increasingly powerless in the regulation and control of the economy and, as such, that political agendas built around the socialisation of the economy are, at best, misguided and, at worst, dangerous. An initial point to make in the refutation of this argument is that it seems obvious enough that different countries have experienced developments in the global economy in different ways. So, for example, developed countries throughout the world have had varied experiences according, for example, to their propensity for investment, the relationships between firms and banking systems, and the degree of protectionism in their economies (Hutton 1996; Gray 1995; Fukuyama 1995). Similarly, rather than simply being held to ransom by transnational corporations, less developed and developing nations can influence the ways in which transnationals operate within their area of jurisdiction depending, for example, on the extent of protection for workers, whether production is solely oriented towards exports, the form of enticements offered and the kinds of company which they wish to attract. Thus the experience of globalisation has varied between Japan and the USA, between India and Latin America, and both between and within the Asian tiger economies (Jordan 1996: 124–5). In this sense the notion that globalisation is a ceaseless and seamless process which negates the attempts of nation states (or blocs of nations) to regulate economies is overly simplistic. Too often it is created as a smokescreen to justify the continued liberalisation of markets.

> The idea of a new, highly-internationalised, virtually uncontrollable global economy based on world market forces has taken root very strongly. It is being used to tell workers and the poor that they must accept whatever is left when their lives and hopes have been sacrificed on the altar of international competitiveness.
>
> (Hirst and Thompson 1996: 48)

Hirst and Thompson provide a rigorous critique of the proponents of the pervasive thesis of globalisation. This thesis suggests that governments are increasingly impotent when it comes to economic policy and, because the success of the economy is held to be the most important indicator (despite the idea that the state is relatively powerless), social policy. Hirst and Thompson suggest that an international economy is not a new phenomenon and that levels of protection or freedom of markets have always fluctuated. Moreover, they argue that the negative extent of capital mobility on jobs and living standards in developed economies is generally overstated and that the necessity of trade means that the model of low-wage, newly industrialising countries continually undercutting Western wage levels is economically unsustainable. Part of the reason for the widespread overestimation of the extent of globalisation, according to Hirst and Thompson, is the myth that the global economy is now governed by a range of footloose transnational corporations when, in fact, these corporations tend to have rather solid bases in the countries in which they are located and rely heavily on sales in home markets or with a relatively small group of trading partners. Thus government decisions are never purely at the behest of foreign transnational corporations, and indeed they may come under just as much pressure from national companies. In this sense 'the image of transnational companies beyond all governance is false' (Hirst and Thompson 1996: 57). Furthermore, Hirst and Thompson argue that the hegemonic position held by world financial markets and the promotion of their values are also not beyond governance – a point that is also raised by Will Hutton (1996) in his argument for the development of a long-termist ethos in the United Kingdom economy.

The most important aspect of the globalisation thesis in terms of the material covered here is the notion that changes in the international economy have escalated competition in labour markets and put paid to

5

the furtherance of governmental social programmes and increased public expenditure on welfare. Hirst and Thompson reject the former on the grounds that it is not international competition that creates low-paid work in developed nations because the low paid in United Kingdom, for example, are not in the same labour markets as the low paid in less developed economies. Thus,

> most unskilled services will never be internationally tradable. This low-wage strategy is best described as seeking competitive advantage through sweating – but it is mad . . . [A] generalised strategy of wage-cutting will depress domestic effective demand, output and employment . . . The sources of such policies are not 'global' pressures, but a mixture of domestic interest groups using this rhetoric to feather their own nests and a failure of nerve by those who should be offering clear alternative policies, a timidity reinforced by the belief in global competitive threats.
>
> (Hirst and Thompson 1996: 60)

According to this argument, the relative depression of wage levels which has been a feature of recent United Kingdom labour markets has actually been harmful for the economy insofar as there are pressures which will result in lower standards of living. Moreover, there is little evidence to suggest that there are actually optimum percentage levels of public expenditure which will improve the economy of any given nation, and several examples of countries in which high percentage levels of public expenditure have not directly impeded the health of the economy, such as Sweden and the Netherlands (Hirst and Thompson 1996: 61–3). Indeed, a strong case can be made for the primacy of social welfare provision in ensuring general welfare which could lead to less rather than more strain on public expenditure generally. Hirst and Thompson also point to a range of issues from poor economic management to tax-cutting, rather than pressure from global markets, as the causes of ideological commitments to lowering public expenditure. Thus there 'is no clear evidence that public expenditure *per se* undermines growth or economic performance' (Hirst and Thompson 1996: 63). This provides impetus for the post-industrial Left which is driven by the economic efficiencies that can derive from universal social and economic policies rather than the knee-jerk rejection of higher public spending as a tool for greater social welfare.

Clearly, the conditions which give rise to post-industrial socialist theory concerning reduced working hours for all and guaranteed income policies are more fully fledged in developed nations rather than those which are less developed, but this does not mean that in the longer term they are not applicable. Indeed, in countries such as South Korea the development process has resulted in ever greater pressure from the workforce for more extensive economic and social protection than has previously been the case. However, the most effective mechanisms for the promotion of rigorous socio-economic provision may lie in international bodies (especially those which trade closely with each other) that may be able to agree central principles which will attach to all their workforces. Ultimately these decisions come down to national governments agreeing to facilitate economic security through international agreements, which corresponds with the advocacy of socio-economic planning that, as we will see, characterises the post-industrial socialist approach (Gorz 1989a, 1994). This needs to take place not just in the national and international domain but also in dialogue with sub-national regions and within the context of a more equitable distribution of global resources between richer and poorer nations. The globalisation thesis does not negate these propositions – indeed, progressive ideas for socio-economic development (which could be arranged around post-industrial socialist principles) 'could be achieved in the near future by more active and co-ordinated policies on the part of the advanced states – what stands in the way is not globalisation but perceptions of "national interest" by key elites' (Hirst and Thompson 1996: 65). On a similar note it is possible to argue that, although globalising tendencies in the economy appear to pressurise governmental expenditure in the public sector, there are also international developments which could lead to more competent social policies if the political and economic will exists.

> Effective social policies allow . . . [welfare] states to throw themselves open to world markets. The tendency is for economic links to grow fastest between countries with similar values, institutional structures and regulatory principles – and in this case the relevant characteristics are political democracy and welfare statism, which provide interdependence and institutional integration with a stable foundation.
>
> (Jordan 1996: 228)

The argument here is not that international bodies and associations of nation states are on the brink of forging radical agreements on social and economic policies – this is patently not the case. However, this does not mean that they are incapable of doing so if the political will existed. It is only through challenging the ubiquitous globalisation thesis that the avenues for change and the constraints on economic policy may be identified.

The economy and ecological politics

The concern with global issues outlined above also feeds into the brand of ecological politics that is encompassed within post-industrial socialism. In maintaining some links with industrial society such as market mechanisms in certain areas where their rationality is appropriate, it should be noted that the post-industrial Left should not be equated with radical political ecology, which would require a more fundamental break with contemporary social organisation. At the same time post-industrial socialism advocates more radical changes to the economy and society than would be the case within mainstream environmentalism (Little 1996: ch. 3; Gorz 1994: 94–5). The main ecological feature of the politics of the post-industrial Left is the notion of self-limitation which has been championed by Gorz (1993). This takes the form of support for an ecologically rational way to produce and consume rather than the promotion of economic rationality which characterises the reproduction of advanced capitalism. Thus Gorz argues that:

> Ecological rationality consists in satisfying material needs in the best way possible with as small a quantity as possible of goods with a high use-value and durability and thus doing so with a minimum of work, capital and natural resources. The quest for maximum economic productivity, by contrast, consists in selling at as high a profit as possible the greatest possible quantity of goods produced with the maximum efficiency, all of which demands a maximization of consumption and needs.
>
> (Gorz 1994: 32)

Where the latter perspective sees this maximum of production and consumption as the central means of maintaining profit margins, ecological rationality sees this approach as characteristic of a wasteful economy which overlooks the necessity of saving resources in order to pursue the process of acquisitively consuming them. Gorz perceives a contradiction in the promotion of economic rationality insofar as it is problematic to suggest that a practice which is ecologically unsustainable should be promoted as being economically rational. In other words, it seems odd to suggest that it is rational to produce and consume goods which will ultimately threaten economic betterment. Thus there would appear to be a necessity to encapsulate both rationalities (economic and ecological) within the post-industrial agenda of working and consuming less. In this sense:

> Ecological modernization requires that investment no longer serve the growth of the economy but its contraction – that is to say, it requires the sphere governed by economic rationality in the modern sense to shrink. There can be no ecological modernization without restricting the dynamic of capitalist accumulation and reducing consumption by self-restraint. The exigencies of ecological modernization coincide with those of a transformed North–South relationship, and with the original aims of socialism.
>
> (Gorz 1994: 33–4)

This passage exemplifies the ideas of the post-industrial Left. They involve strict regulation of the economy and a limitation of the spheres of society in which economic rationality is allowed to dominate. At the same time this concern with ecological politics is accompanied by a recognition of the problems and inequalities between the developed and less developed world which are exacerbated by our failure to deal with the issues which emanate from the global economy. Fusing these perspectives together we have an undoubtedly socialist theory which is informed by ecological rationality and opposed to regional, national and global inequalities.

A central strategy in tackling the organisation of society around economic rationality is opposition to an economy which allows what Beck refers to as 'the new industrial double income' (Beck 1995: 138-9). By this he means the process whereby some businesses (such as large chemical companies) profit from both ecological pollution and environmental campaigns to maintain ecological protection. Companies can produce goods in an environmentally damaging way which increases hazards and risks (Beck 1992) and at the same time other companies (or branches of the same corporation) may profit from producing antidotes to 'protect' against the hazards that are being manufactured. When it comes to the environment, advanced capitalist societies, rather than working to minimise ecological degradation, are actively engaged in a process whereby the economy self-referentially produces ever more problems which necessitate rectification. This rectification takes the form of further economic activity guided by the rationality of growth, accumulation and profit. Ultimately the rationality behind this process is difficult to identify. Is it rational to desolate social and ecological organisation in the interest of economic logic and reproduction? Would not the rational approach be to minimise the production of hazards and risks, thereby minimising the need to protect against them? In short, a society organised around eco-social politics should choose to limit the scope of economic activity rather than reproduce modern economies which subsume ever greater spheres of social and ecological life in the name of progress. For Beck, the challenge for modernist politics is to formulate 'as a social movement and political force against industrial fictions and narrow-mindedness. It is not the end of the Enlightenment, but its deployment against industrial society here and now, that is on today's agenda'(Beck 1995: 183). The self-limitation philosophy of post-industrial socialism is based on a rejection of the logic of industrialism whereby ever-increasing needs are created by the system itself, which increases the need for further production despite the fact that it may have a knock-on effect creating new dangers and reproducing old problems. Self-limitation as part of a political programme is only feasible, though, if economic arrangements are informed by ecological rationality. Governed by ecological rationality, the economy could be stabilised, and markets, which are fragile in contemporary 'risk societies', could be strictly and more effectively regulated, which should provide greater security for individuals working within them.[1] In Gorz's words:

> The ecological approach . . . involves a paradigm shift, which may be summarised in the slogan 'less but better'. It aims to reduce the sphere in which economic rationality and commodity exchanges apply, and to subordinate it to non-quantifiable societal and cultural ends and to the free development of individuals.
>
> (Gorz 1994: 95)

A Left-libertarian philosophy

The other definitional dimension of the post-industrial Left approach, to go along with the notions of a socialised economy and ecological rationality, is the prioritisation of individual autonomy (which has often been opposed as a foundational principle in socialist debates). As such it puts substantial emphasis on the empowerment of individuals to self-determine their activities to the greatest and most equitable extent. To this extent post-industrial socialism is a form of Left-libertarianism because it highlights the importance of autonomy for real human freedom.[2] This differs from right-wing libertarianism which promotes a form of individual autonomy which is centred on formalistic, rights-based negative freedoms. However, unlike 'formal freedom . . . real freedom is not only a matter of having the right to do what one might want to do, but also a matter of having the means for doing it' (Van

Parijs 1995: 4). This primacy of properly resourced individual autonomy for the Left is reinforced by Conrad Lodziak:

> Limited resources imply limited opportunities for autonomy. But the exercise of autonomy also involves an autonomous individual. Autonomous individuals are not born autonomous. Rather the autonomous person is an achievement, it is a product of how we develop . . . What the individual does have is a capacity for autonomy. And there is no reason, at least no valid reason, to suppose that some individuals are born with a greater capacity for autonomy than others . . . The question arises as to whether or not capitalist societies are producing individuals with an insufficiently developed autonomy to withstand the drift into identity crisis. The answers to this question are of vital importance to the Left simply because emancipatory social change involves autonomous agents with a commitment to expanding the sphere of autonomy for everyone.
>
> (Lodziak 1995: 85)

As such the prioritisation of individual autonomy is not something that can be realised in social conditions which do not understand the necessity of creating maximal opportunities for autonomy for all. This goes far beyond the limited conception of individual freedom that prevails in advanced capitalism where it is largely understood in the context of economic activity. For the post-industrial Left, autonomous individuals should have the opportunity to exercise maximal self-determination in all spheres of life regardless of imposed economic imperatives. This is the foundation of Lodziak's theory of a culture of opposition which he believes could be engendered by *an expansion of the sphere in which autonomy is the guiding principle* – that is, the sphere which is not governed by economic necessity or other bonds of necessity such as self-maintenance. Moreover, the expansion of autonomy is to be collective in the senses that the experience of autonomy is to be spread throughout society and that the expansion of autonomy will move individuals away from the destructive route of privatism and towards co-operative associations of interest which help to express collective self-determination. This is not a purely theoretical proposition. Lodziak, following Gorz, suggests that political decisions must be made to provide facilities on a local basis to enable individuals to pursue self-determined and collective goals, and policies must be formulated in which non-market bodies and communities are allowed to develop without direct control by the state or the irrational forces of market mechanisms (Lodziak 1995: 110–11).

11

The post-industrial Left, then, maintains a resource-based dimension in the conceptualisation of freedom in society. Van Parijs notes how there is a contradiction in the supposition that a free society entails freedom for the individuals within that society. Thus the notion that a society as a whole might be free to determine organisation without coercion from other societies does not necessarily mean that citizens of that society will also be emancipated. In this sense it is quite possible that there might actually be some conflict between a totally free society and the freedom of the people therein (such as in the example of conscription): 'Maximal freedom for society as a whole is bound to clash with the maximal freedom of its individual members' (Van Parijs 1995: 16). How, then, should Left-libertarians conceptualise freedom within their commitment to maximum resourced autonomy? The answer lies in further examining the meaning of the relationship between free individuals and the free society. In this sense freedom is not just something which we formally have or do not have but an entity which we experience within a social context. Thus individual freedom can only be meaningfully experienced within a society which promotes maximal freedom for all (which will involve some limitation of pure individual freedoms as is the case with all modern societies). Thus Van Parijs states that 'a free society . . . [is] a society whose members are all free or as free as possible' (Van Parijs 1995: 20). In this sense Left-libertarians can argue that maximal self-ownership is the rationale behind their preferred mode of social organisation but that there will always be some 'institutional restrictions' on freedoms in modern societies. Within the post-industrial socialist perspective these restrictions would be manifest in reduced working hours for all and a form of guaranteed income (which will be explained in more detail later in the book). This feeds into what Van Parijs terms 'real freedom' which, in contrast to the negative rights-based freedom of right-wing libertarianism, involves not only rights-based security and self-ownership but resourced opportunities to exercise self-determination.[3] Thus,

> real-libertarianism can be viewed, along with other left-liberal
> positions, as an attempt to articulate the importance we ascribe
> to liberty, equality, and efficiency. Liberty comes in through the
> postulate of neutrality, through the constraint of self-ownership
> (or fundamental liberties and the like), and through a concern,
> not directly with people's happiness itself, but with the means
> required to pursue it.
>
> (Van Parijs 1995: 28)

This feeds into the post-industrial socialist position on welfare. In contrast to the statist paternalism of the social democratic perspective, it is not to be conceived as something which is doled out by the state to the needy or to those who cannot satisfy needs through economic activity as long as they fulfil eligibility criteria that correspond with preordained social values. Rather, welfare is something a society has as a whole – it is akin to the distribution of betterment throughout a society. Social welfare, then, entails everyone in a society contributing to the common good and, as a result, everyone should have a reasonable expectation to be allowed to a share in it. This involves the protection of citizens from the vicissitudes of market-based society and the facilitation of participation by citizens rather than social exclusion. As will become clear in the course of the book this is a task which has not been tackled sufficiently by the social democratic welfare state (in all its variants). In this vein Kallscheuer argues that: 'Regulation by the social state – necessary as it may be for the want of anything better – creates no social solidarity, but compensates for social decay, arising from (and constantly reproduced by) "asocial social-ization" in the world of consumption' (Kallscheuer 1994: 120).

A redefined socialism must develop a coherent position on welfare which will reiterate the values of solidarity and social justice within the context of Left-libertarianism. This involves the organisation of society in such a way that all individuals are given meaningful choices about the blend of activities in which they spend their time and recognise a respon-sibility to facilitate the expansion of these choices for all. In this sense: 'Autonomy . . . implies the social integration of individuals. Socially-integrated conduct is self-regulated by individuals who co-ordinate the attainment of common goals by consensus' (Bowring 1996: 103). This social dimension of developed autonomy should provide further impetus for individuals to recognise the eco-social constraints on human action which need to be understood both collectively and individually. Thus, for Gorz, 'self-limitation remains the only non-authoritarian, democratic way towards an eco-compatible industrial civilization' (Gorz 1993: 64). In turn, it is the process of emancipating human time and thereby providing more autonomous choices which will enable individuals (and the collec-tive units of which they are a part) to lead a less wasteful existence and embrace the principles of self-limitation. This is the junction at which post-industrial socialism and Left-libertarian philosophy meet. To quote Lodziak:

> The expansion of the sphere of autonomy involves an increase in resourced time for everyone in social conditions conducive to the exercise of individual and collective autonomy. The most appropriate vehicle for bringing about an increase in resourced

POST-INDUSTRIAL SOCIALISM

time is an emancipatory politics of time in conjunction with a
politics of collective resources. The social conditions which best
facilitate the exercise of autonomy are what I refer to as a culture for autonomy – a culture grounded in relations
characterised by genuine concern for the other, equality, mutual
trust and co-operation, and involving the practical enactment of
individual and community-based autonomous projects.

(Lodziak 1995: 117–18)

Having outlined the theoretical impetus behind post-industrial socialism it is important to identify where it stands in relation to other
developments in socialist thought and different interpretations of the
'post-industrialisation' of the economy. From there it will be possible to
highlight potential options in social and economic policies which correspond with the political perspective of the post-industrial Left.

1

EXPLORING POST-INDUSTRIAL SOCIALISM

Since the 1960s there has been a growth in literature questioning the continuing nature of industrialism and the potential advent of a post-industrial society. Originally this perspective gained most influence in neo-pluralist circles in the USA, although it was also inspired by the rise of a variety of social movements in the late 1960s (Dunleavy and O'Leary 1987: 290–2). This development has been accompanied more recently by proclamations that Western capitalism has moved variously from Fordism to post-Fordism (Amin 1994b), from modernity to post-modernity or into the age of McDonaldisation (Ritzer 1993). The 1990s have also witnessed new literature which accepts that post-industrial societies have now emerged (Esping-Andersen 1991, 1993; Clement and Myles 1994).

This chapter will evaluate these approaches and highlight the differences between them and the notion of post-industrial socialism. The analysis of the latter perspective will demonstrate that post-industrial society has not yet developed and that, for the Left, post-industrialism will be evident only with an end to 'work-based society'. Thus post-industrial socialism contends that a genuinely post-industrial society cannot be founded upon the principle that individuals should spend a large portion of their time in work for wages. Moreover, I will argue that a mature post-industrial society will be one in which the work that is available is shared around more equitably than is presently the case. This would allow individuals to spend time engaging in other self-determined activities and performing unpaid or voluntary work in their communities (Gorz 1989a, 1994). This differs considerably from the orthodox perspective that post-industrialism is characterised by the advent of 'the information society' (Kumar 1995: ch. 2).

Clearly, the growth of flexible working and the end of full (male) employment have signalled enormous changes in the structures of labour markets across a wide variety of industries (including many in the service sector) and in a range of developed nations including the

USA, Germany and Japan (Currie 1995: 67–9). However, in this chapter I shall contend that changes in labour markets do not by themselves signify a qualitative change to an era of post-industrialism or, for that matter, post-Fordism. The main feature of this argument is that there is a difference between the concept of the post-industrial economy and the notion of post-industrial society and that the latter is not necessarily technologically determined by the former. In this sense 'shifts in the character and distribution of work *could* open up new possibilities for creating a more civilized society of genuine abundance; they could also drive us into ever greater social insecurity, deprivation, and conflict' (Currie 1995: 65). For the post-industrial Left, it is the latter which has been the outcome of changes in the new economy. In other words, a post-industrial society has not evolved alongside the embryonic post-industrial economy. This contradicts the ideas of Therborn, who argues that the 'politico-economic changes of the past two decades have had the character of an epochal transition – the culmination of industrial society and industrial class politics and the emerging of a postindustrial society' (Therborn 1991: 101). As should become clear, the decline of central features of industrialism does not mean that we have entered into a post-industrial society. Initially, though, it is important to evaluate the relationship between industrialism and post-industrialism and to outline a socialist perspective on developments in industrial capitalism.

Socialism and post-industrialism

One of the first major contributions to the debate on post-industrialism emanated from Daniel Bell with the publication of *The Coming of Post-Industrial Society* in 1973 in which he argued that changes in class structure and declining organised labour had negated Marxist visions of social change.[1] Rather, he looked positively towards a future post-industrial society in which affluent consumers would exist in a high-technology, service-based economy and knowledge-based society. The subtitle to the book, 'A Venture in Social Forecasting', is pertinent because it indicates that Bell was aware of the deep and resilient embeddedness of structures of industrialism in social and economic life in the early 1970s. What is at stake for the post-industrial Left is whether the forecast of increasing affluence has taken place in a substantive way in the intervening years since Bell's book. Clearly, the tertiary sector has grown as Bell believed it would (as have the other non-manufacturing sectors of the economy which he identified) but 'in contrast to Bell's thesis, low-status blue collar and service occupations show no signs of disappearing' (Ritzer 1993: 153). This is the case not only in Western capitalist nations but must also be located within the context of the growth of manufacturing and secondary industry in less developed parts of the world (Calinicos 1989: 125). Moreover, Bell's notion of increasing affluence seriously underestimates the distinction between the overall wealth in advanced capitalism (which may be very narrowly distributed) and the lived experience of the mass of individuals who suffer from the social inequalities, insecurity and marginalisation which characterise contemporary capitalist societies. To this extent, Lodziak argues that 'theorists of the post-industrial society embrace a flawed conception of power which enables them to misconstrue the relation between the social totality and the individual' (Lodziak 1986: 193).

The critique of mainstream post-industrialism

Undoubtedly much has changed in the structures of labour markets since Bell's social forecast first appeared and this has had profound effects on social organisation. However, it is highly debatable whether these changes can be equated with any kind of mature post-industrialism. For instance, Bell was far too quick to equate the downfall of trade unionism with the decline of work as a central issue in the organisation of capitalist societies when he suggested that 'the crucial fact is that the "labor issue" *qua* labor is no longer central, nor does it have the sociological and cultural weight to polarize all other issues along that axis' (Bell 1973: 164). In this suggestion Bell confuses the importance of the issue of work (and the lack thereof) with the decline of organised labour. On the contrary, I would argue that the decline of trade unions has (not surprisingly) taken place alongside – and as a result of – the *increased* centrality of work as a key category in social life. In other words, as work becomes increasingly less available so the role of trade unions becomes less central while, at the same time, the possession of work becomes an ever more important mode of social inclusion and citizenship. In this sense organised labour is at its strongest when there is a highly ordered and disciplined labour market in which there is a clear constituency for trade unions to represent. However, the labour market of today is flexible, transitory and disorganised, with a strong growth of part-time and non-unionised labour, often in the service sector. In this scenario work and unemployment are increasingly important as harbingers of a post-Marshallian economic citizenship (which will be identified here as the right to meaningful work *and* the right to an income independent of a direct work requirement), whereas the representation of workers through trade unionism becomes increasingly tenuous.

The rhetoric of mainstream advocates of the post-industrial society looks all the more misguided as contemporary capitalist societies witness the new divisions in labour markets between core and peripheral work-ers and non-workers. These new divisions result in a situation whereby much new work is in the tertiary sector which is frequently lowly paid with little job-security and yet simultaneously a large number of individ-uals remain marginalised from the economy (and society as a whole) through the absence of sufficient jobs. This explains why many on the Left have been sceptical of any attempt to embrace post-industrialism because it does little to challenge the logic of capital accumulation or the fragmentation of labour markets. Thus Wilde contends that 'develop-ments in the forces of production and alterations in the specific forms of production relations do not constitute a departure from the logic of the capital accumulation process' (Wilde 1994: 100).[2] From this perspec-tive the increasing fragmentation of labour markets should not be viewed as the inevitable result of the post-industrialisation of the econ-omy but rather as the outcome of neo-liberal policies which prioritise 'efficiency' in labour markets and the leanest possible labour force. Moreover, Lee argues that the divisions in labour markets are produced by the primacy of 'efficiency' (which is a key by-product of industrialism rather than post-industrialism) and as a result contemporary times should not be dubbed 'post-industrial' but 'rather the era of mass per-manent unemployment' (Lee 1993: 108).

Towards a progressive vision of post-industrialism

Lee correctly identifies that post-industrial visions of highly technologi-cal, service economies in which affluent consumers abound cannot be equated with contemporary Western capitalism, but fails to acknowledge that post-industrialism can also exist in a more radical format than the type of 'conservative' social forecast propounded by Bell. Drawing on the work of Michael Marien, Dobson outlines differences between what he calls 'dominant post-industrialism' which is seen as 'an affluent, techno-logical, service society' and more progressive visions of post-industrialism inspired by political ecology (Dobson 1990: 5–7). It is this kind of radical post-industrialism which is the main concern here, although the intel-lectual heritage of the key ideas involved can just as easily be attributed to what Offe (1992: 700) calls the 'left-libertarian' ideological orientation as to political ecology. André Gorz points to the type of policies which the Left, informed by radical anthropocentric environmentalism, should follow in the development of post-industrial socialism:

> To exist politically, an ecological Left has, consequently, an urgent need for *mediations* between the existing industrial

system, its wage-workers and its jobs, on the one hand, and, on the other, post-industrial forms of society which comply both with ecological demands and with individuals' aspirations to liberate themselves *from* work as it exists and find *in* work as great a potential for self-determination as possible. We have to start out from what work *is* and what it really means today in order to transform it, reduce it, and expand the scope for autonomous activities, production for one's own use and self-realization for everyone.

(Gorz 1994: 64)

Clearly, then, for radical post-industrialists, a post-industrial society requires qualitative societal changes as well as alterations in the mode of production. While the latter does have a wide and powerful influence on social and economic life, it does not necessarily define social relations. Thus, whilst the move towards a service-based economy – the process of tertiarisation – is taking place in Western capitalism, attitudes towards work and employment have not altered at a similar pace. In other words, moves towards a redefinition of the way we work have not been accompanied by a recognition that there is a possibility that this redefinition could facilitate an understanding that the prospect of 'the end of work-based society', that is, genuine post-industrialism, could come on to the agenda. If this scenario is valid – and the pace of technological change suggests that it could be – then, as Gorz points out, dialogue on a social level is necessary to prepare and plan for the future. On a similar note, Sherman argues that:

The new industrial revolution is different from the first in that we are partially aware of what is happening . . . Technology is changing, employment is changing, products and services are changing – but the one key change has not occurred. As happened eventually in the course of the nineteenth century, we need a revolution in attitudes to match that in industry.

(Sherman 1986: 276)

Progress towards a post-industrial society, therefore, requires more than *changes to the kind of work we perform*. It necessitates debate and planning about how to translate changes in working patterns into the *organisation of society and everyday life* through legislation to lessen the centrality of work (Currie 1995: 75). A post-industrial society cannot be deterministically fashioned by an increase in employment in the service sector of the economy, it can only be created by investigating the nature of the new economy and understanding the opportunities that it generates and then changing social organisation appropriately. Post-industrialism has hitherto been characterised by the likes of Bell as the advent of a knowledge-based society without recognising that knowledge can be restricted to a rather small section of society. Thus the forces of post-industrialism in the economy are open to manipulation and can be extremely divisive when applied to society in general. Obviously, socialist post-industrialism must aim to create a society in which divisions and inequalities are minimised. This has not been the case with the new economy which has encouraged social polarisation and marginalisation for many who do not benefit from flexible labour markets. Thus post-industrial socialism opposes the technological determinism employed as much by Bell as by the Marxists he attempted to negate (Clement and Myles 1994: 26–7). Rather, post-industrial socialism opens up possibilities for democratic dialogue between employers and employees, the state and local communities and institutions of civil society, individuals and their communities, and women and men (Gorz 1982: 85-7). This kind of dialogue is designed to encourage debate about work and human activity in general and to negotiate, among other things, how that work is going to be distributed.

Post-industrialism and the economy

Clearly, post-industrial socialism is still in its infancy as a political project but it is also an ambitious project which asks questions of the very nature of democracy and advanced capitalism. It is concerned with challenging the nature of changes in the economy and their effects on social realities. In this sense it should not be confused with contemporary literature which confuses moves towards post-industrial economies with the altogether different notion of post-industrial societies (Clement and Myles 1994; Esping-Andersen 1993, 1994). Post-industrial socialism also stands in contrast to those who focus on issues relating to post-industrialism and class mobility. Gershuny, for instance, concentrates on occupational mobility and employs empirical data to demonstrate relatively high mobility into and out of 'low-level service occupations' (Gershuny 1993: 139). This does not mean that these jobs do not exist in large numbers, it merely (and not surprisingly) indicates that people change jobs with increased frequency in the new economy. Gershuny's evidence says little about unemployment and he openly admits that, while the United Kingdom may not have a steady group of individuals who are part of a low-level service-related class, it may well be a dualistic society. It is precisely this kind of dualised and polarised society that post-industrial socialism stands against. Gershuny's line of thought is reflected by Blossfeld, Giannelli and Mayer, who argue that there is high mobility between categories of unskilled employment in Germany, suggesting that 'unskilled service jobs can be regarded as a "collecting vessel" for redundant manual workers' (Blossfeld *et al.* 1993: 134). The argument against a new post-industrial service class is continued by Jacobs who states that 'the good news is that the bottom of the post-industrial society is far from closed . . . the bad news is that the economic distance from bottom to top is growing' (Jacobs 1993: 223). Similarly Myles, Picot and Wannell, in celebrating mobility from low-level service employment in Canada, state that: 'Occupational skill levels have risen over the postwar period, but despite rising skill levels, low-wage employment has grown faster than average or high-paying jobs' (Myles *et al.* 1993: 189).

All of the authors above concentrate on the belief that there is not a new class created by post-industrial economies and at the same time all admit that there is increased social polarisation. The notion that there is mobility within different categories of low-level employment does not negate the post-industrial socialist view that polarisation and marginalisation are increasing as a result of the new economy. Moreover, if that economy determines society at the moment, then it is creating social fragmentation rather than an affluent, knowledge-based society. This does not mean that this situation is the inevitable result of a post-industrial economy, rather post-industrial socialists believe that society can be improved along with the new economy if the political will to do so exists. Yet many analysts of post-industrialism continue to suggest that 'the real polarization that does exist applies . . . not to skills but to the attributes of jobs' while simultaneously noting that 'inequalities of earnings, and the proportion of people in precarious jobs have risen sharply. The unskilled and new labour-force entrants are the two groups that have been most severely affected' (Esping-Andersen 1994: 175–6). This would appear to suggest that polarisation with regards to skills is likely to increase. If more jobs are becoming precarious and insecure, it seems unlikely that the contemporary 'post-industrial' economies in the West will close the deficit between the securely employed and the growing group living in insecurity.[3]

For post-industrial socialists, the economy needs to be controlled and subject to planning to eradicate the insecurity and inequalities that it produces at the moment. This presupposes a radical reappraisal of the way in which governments (attempt to) manage their economies. Planning is anathema to most political and economic thinking in contemporary times, although clearly governments do operate economic plans on a regular basis. The annual budget in the United Kingdom, for instance, is an examination of previous economic performance and a projection of economic planning for the future (for example, plans to cut public spending). Similarly, all companies operate on the basis of economic planning to survive (Gorz 1992). This is not to say that planning is always accurate and reliable, but it does (by necessity) take place. Clarification and democratisation of economic planning is important for post-industrial socialism because, like all proposals aimed at regenerating socialism, it must outline what role market mechanisms will play in the socialist alternative to current arrangements. Moreover, it needs to be explicit about the means of developing a transparent economic system which must be coupled with a more thorough understanding of the relationship between social and economic policy (which will be analysed towards the end of this book).

A role for markets?

A variety of literature from the Left has been characterised in recent times by the level of attention given to 'the market'. Of course, it is not an issue that socialists have ever been reticent about, but the post-industrial Left is explicitly concerned with deciding what role the market will have in a socialist society as opposed to the tendency to reject all the workings of the market as antithetical to socialist objectives. In the contemporary era the most influential body of work in the area has been the resurgence of interest in market socialism (Roemer 1994; Le Grand and Estrin 1989; Pierson 1995)[4] but interesting contributions to the debate over the role of market mechanisms have also emanated from post-industrialist socialists such as Gorz (1989b) and, of course, elements within socialist and social democratic parties in Europe (Brown 1994). This is not to say that all of the Left now embraces a role for markets in a socialist society, but even so-called 'utopian' writers such as Gorz are prepared to envisage an appropriate location for market rationality in a socialist alternative to contemporary capitalism.

It is important to note that most work emanating from the Left on markets begins from a critical view of the operation of markets in contemporary capitalism. These criticisms range from the inability of the market to meet needs, particularly those of the worst-off members of society (Sherman 1986: 172), the short-termism of market rationality and the incompatibility with sustainability (Dobson 1990: 126), the inability of the market to provide public goods (Doyal and Gough 1991: 292), the generation of unequal welfare outcomes (Pierson 1991: 217–18) and the tendency of markets to undermine citizenship and create individual consumers (Bauman 1987: 188–9). These sentiments are clearly echoed by Bankowski, who suggests that 'markets encourage greed instead of self-lessness. Indifference to one's neighbour rather than concern. Selfishness and avarice is promoted to the level of a virtue' (Bankowski 1993: 92). Even commentators whose aspirations are not particularly socialistic note the danger of founding social principles in the market. For instance, Handy states that 'markets do not look much beyond tomorrow, or at least next year. Markets are inherently selfish, disinclined to make investments whose outcomes cannot be precisely predicted or whose benefits cannot be claimed in advance' (Handy 1990: 207). Clearly, then, there is plenty of opposition to markets as they operate currently from a range of ideological viewpoints despite the hegemonic status attached to market mechanisms in recent years, especially in welfare debates. What functions, then, are there for market mechanisms in a socialist society? There are three main perspectives on this question holding particular sway in contemporary debates: market socialism; socialism with markets; and the social democratic social market.

Three perspectives on markets

While market socialism can be connected concretely with the economies of some nations in Central and Eastern Europe (Pierson 1995; Little 1996), the intention here is to analyse the resurgence of market socialism which has emerged and strengthened since the 1980s. The basis of this perspective is that the market is not inherently a feature of capitalism and that some of the 'virtues' of the market such as efficiency could be usefully employed in a socialist society. Vincent states that 'for market socialists, capitalism may be impossible without markets, but markets can function without capitalism' (Vincent 1992: 95). However, market socialism is not really concerned with replacing capitalism, rather it is a doctrine concerned with humanising the economic system and regulating it to prevent the excesses which are linked to the operation of markets in contemporary capitalism. It can also be linked to the notion of stakeholder capitalism in which individuals hold a stake in the economy through industrial democracy and co-operative decision-making in the firms in which they are employed. For Tomlinson, though, market socialism equates too closely with New Right glorification of the market. He chastises Miller and Estrin (1986) for providing 'a gloss on a neo-Hayekian celebration of the market in a manner wholly incompatible with socialist objectives' (Tomlinson 1990: 32). This thesis of incompatibility is continued by Pierson, who accuses market socialists of abandoning 'traditional socialist baggage' (Pierson 1995: 86). To what extent, then, can such a system be regarded as socialist? According to

23

Baker, 'the system would be socialist, because firms would be worker-managed, the major means of production would be socially owned, and the overall shape and direction of the economy would be democratically planned' (Baker 1987: 107).

However, there is a substantial body of work which suggests that workers' self-management is nothing more than a transitional phase in gradualist socialist programmes rather than a developed form of socialism in itself (Little 1996: ch. 2). From this perspective self-management within market socialism does little to challenge the pervasiveness of the economic rationality of the market in every sphere of everyday life. Most market socialists too readily assume that markets can be easily detached from capitalist rationality – a claim that many Marxists (and the New Right, for that matter) would not accept. Indeed, Pierson notes several reasons why socialists and the New Right regard market socialism as a contradiction in terms (Pierson 1995: 111–35; Harrington 1993: 247). Market socialism rests upon the idea that markets do not have their own rationality as such but that they are currently imbued with the values of capitalism and could just as easily be made to operate along socialist lines. An example of this tendency is Miller's claim that 'where community exists . . . the presence of markets need not destroy it' (Miller 1992: 85). As Miller suggests that there is no conflict of interests between the values of community and the rationality of the market, he appears to believe that the market is a neutral mechanism in some way. However, he does not recognise that markets may have their own economic rationality even if they are liberated from acting towards capitalist ends (Gorz 1989a). Moreover, market socialism tends to revert to the perspective that we face a stark alternative between the market and centralised state planning. For this reason Tomlinson claims that 'market socialism is a profoundly conservative notion . . . that can lead socialism nowhere helpful' (Tomlinson 1990: 45). He also takes market socialists to task for the essentialisation of the notion of the market:

> There is no such thing as 'the market', but only markets, whose effects are determined by the agents who operate in them, their forms of calculation, their relation to other agents, and the legal and moral (as Hayek himself emphasises) framework in which they operate.
>
> (Tomlinson 1990: 43)

This does not mean that there is not necessarily a role for markets in socialist debates. Pierson and Tomlinson both argue that the problem with market socialism is that the emphasis is quite frequently placed more on the market element of the equation than on socialism. However, in line with the second perspective on markets mentioned above, they both state that there might be greater value in the notion of 'socialism with markets'. Tomlinson points out a line of work in the socialist tradition which has debated potential roles for markets. He prefers (following Alec Nove) a socialist system founded on a range of principles which are provided by a range of mechanisms including markets and planning. What this perspective appears to underestimate is that these mechanisms are not necessarily value-free and that they are employed because of different types of rationality driving them. Thus it is not sufficient to advocate a mixture of planning and markets without intimating which areas are to be subject to which mechanism.[5] However, it is in keeping with the general thrust of post-industrial socialism that 'discussion of markets can proceed on the basis that they are possible tools that may (or may not) advance these [socialist] principles in specific institutional contexts' (Tomlinson 1990: 34).

In the debate over the role of markets it is interesting to note that most conceptions of post-industrialism do envisage some kind of knowledge-society. Markets, on the other hand, do not currently operate towards the dissemination of knowledge. Rather, as Michael Harrington notes, 'markets . . . often function to obscure information rather then providing it. Therefore it is necessary to talk about "socialising" the market . . . to provide consumers with objective knowledge for their choices' (Harrington 1993: 246–7). This is broadly in line with the post-industrial socialist approach to organisation of markets and Harrington provides a succinct analysis of the way forward:

> The aim . . . is a socialism that makes markets a tool of its non-market purposes. And it is not totally utopian for the new socialists to argue that, in liberating markets from the capitalist context that frustrates their virtues, the visible hand can use the invisible hand for its own purposes.
>
> (Harrington 1993: 247)

Before concluding this section with a discussion of post-industrial socialism and market mechanisms, it is important to evaluate the third of the dominant perspectives in contemporary political debates – that of the social democratic Left. Some recent contributions to mainstream debates have begun to embrace the notion of the social market in a restatement of the values of social democracy and the mixed economy (Rocard 1994; Hutton 1994, 1996). The notion of a social market economy, particularly applicable to West German social democracy in the post-war years, is centred upon economic growth and full employment which provide for a relatively inexpensive welfare regime (based on insurance principles in the West German case). This is problematic for post-industrial socialism because of the reliance on economic growth without understanding the ecological implications of unrestrained growth and the presentation of full employment as the ultimate desirable goal (Harrington 1993: 106).

Advocates of the social market, such as Rocard, suggest that the market is inescapable and ubiquitous. The role of the state becomes increasingly regulatory, overseeing the distribution of resources and ensuring that the liberalised market economy does not cause too much inequality. Rocard, unlike some of the advocates of market socialism, realises that the market is not value-free – indeed, he suggests that it can have pernicious effects:

> We need a market economy, but creating a society of social solidarity means more than a free market. By definition, the effects of markets increase inequalities. The market creates growing disequilibria. It encourages not only concentration of consumption but concentration in the means of production. A society of solidarity in a market economy requires a public authority with the responsibility to preserve social cohesion.
>
> (Rocard 1994: 154)

So much for Miller's argument presented above that the market does not have conflicting values with community. Here Rocard, as fervent a supporter of the potential of markets as Miller, argues that markets *by definition* create inequalities. Surely Miller would not suggest that communitarian socialism can be created by a mechanism which increases inequality (Hughes and Little 1996). Again Miller's contention that the market is in some way neutral looks highly questionable. As far as Rocard is concerned, his belief in the necessity of the market and the ability of the state to regulate it effectively is a classic statement of contemporary European social democracy but, as Hutton suggests, this is overly optimistic and yields far too much ground to right-wing economics (Hutton 1994). Moreover, there are further problems with the social market approach, such as the overreliance on an anachronistic workerism and the inability to countenance anything other than orthodox approaches to the economy. Similarly, though, Hutton's restatement of 'why Keynesian economics is best' is an inherently industrialist and workerist approach to economic problems because it is also inherently reliant on economic growth as part of the panacea to cure our economic ills. Despite his advocacy of long-termism in economic policy, he does not extend that ethos to take account of environmental reasons for limiting economic growth and the operation of market mechanisms (Hutton 1996).

Post-industrial socialism and markets

The post-industrial socialist perspective on markets has much in common with the 'socialism with markets' approach, except that it is much more rigorous in delineating the role of markets and the areas of society in which they would be permitted to operate. The most rigorous thinker in this area is André Gorz, who has proposed a number of radical reforms to diminish the sphere of influence in which markets would work while simultaneously outlining why markets cannot be abolished.[6] Gorz is keen to outline the difference between markets and market mechanisms on one hand and 'the market' or the market economy on the other:

> [Y]ou can have commodity production and exchange, markets and market mechanisms without having a market economy. A market economy is one where prices are determined by the so-called law of supply and demand, both of which are supposed to adjust freely to each other.
>
> (Gorz 1989b: 29–30)

In other words, the post-industrial Left need not spend futile time wishing away the need for markets or embracing them wholeheartedly as the key foundation for economic and social organisation. If we can allocate appropriate spaces for market mechanisms in the domain of the economy, then we can organise the rest of society along other principles. This is the key to differentiating between markets and the market economy. For Gorz, it is erroneous to refer to the market economy as central to modern societies anyway, as none of them are really regulated by the law of supply and demand:

> In all the industrial nations, the relative price of goods and services are regulated by the state; if they weren't, society wouldn't be viable. Everything that's vital is subsidized: agricultural production, housing, health, transport, education, libraries, research, museums, theatres, and so on. And the rest is taxed to varying degrees by a system of VAT or specific taxes . . . The more extensive the sphere of commodity relations, the more the state has to intervene in the market mechanisms to correct and regulate their functioning. The fact is that the market is, by definition, the outcome of the activities of individuals each pursuing

his or her own immediate interests. Thus a higher authority, the
state, is required to take responsibility for defending the general
interest, including the existence of a market system.

(Gorz 1994: 82–3)

The post-industrial socialist view on markets, then, is that they should
remain but they should be restricted to areas where economic rationality
is appropriate. Of course, this necessitates a definition of economic rationality and an indication of where that rationality lies. Moreover, we need
to outline the differences between socialist economic rationality and that
of classical economics. Hutton provides a powerful critique of economic
rationality in free market theory by arguing that individuals are social
beings who undertake work not only for wages but also for social interaction and self-esteem. Thus the reason why people work is not just to
provide resources for consumption (Lane 1991). From this perspective
Hutton argues that 'this does not mean that men and women are indif-
ferent to what they earn – but the supposed free market calculus that they
work up to the exact moment when the disutility of working offsets the
loss of utility from leisure fails to capture the nature of the bargain over
work' (Hutton 1996: 231). On this basis Hutton concludes that we cannot
be altogether rational about the market because there will always be
uncertainty about market outcomes.

Hutton's critique of classical economics is a valuable negation of the
propagation of free market ideas. However, it is problematic from the
post-industrial socialist perspective because it rests heavily on the notion
that markets are difficult to interpret rationally. This may well be the case
but it does not assist socialists who seek to delineate a sphere for the
market. Is it possible, then, to impart a version of economic rationality
which has utility for the post-industrial Left? Gorz offers a version which
proceeds from a different starting point from Hutton. The former
believes that if we can decide what work is economically rational, then
economic and social policy can be geared towards reducing working
hours and spreading economically rational work out more equitably.
Thus he is attempting to outline what should be performed rationally
within markets which is different from Hutton's approach which centres
on economic rationality *of the market*. Where the former perspective is
designed to provide a basis for the limitation of markets, the latter
accepts that they are to hold a powerful role. Gorz believes that:

Actions are economically rational in so far as they aim at the
maximization of productivity. But this becomes possible only
on two conditions: (1) Labour has to be separated from the

28

personal singularity of the labourer and must be expressed as a calculable and measurable quantity; and (2) The economic goal of the maximization of productivity cannot be subordinated to any non-economic social, cultural or religious goals; it must be pursued ruthlessly.

(Gorz 1994: 68)

This gives a very different meaning to economic rationality from Hutton's definition. It presents a radical method of deciding which work should be performed in what Gorz calls the macro-social sphere where markets may well be the most efficient and effective methods of ensuring the maximisation of productivity. In this scenario the macro-social sphere becomes the domain of work-for-wages which Gorz, along with Hutton and Lane believes, is essential for self-esteem and self-development. If shared around equally this work becomes a central tenet of what I have referred to as economic citizenship. The idea of sharing this work around more equitably would necessitate a policy of reduced working hours for everyone. This is a central plank of post-industrial socialist thinking because it signals the end of 'work-based society' in which everyone has to compete for employment which is rationed between those in full-time employment and those who either work for wages part time, irregularly or not at all. In Gorz's theory the delineation of the macro-social sphere and the mechanisms which would operate therein would allow us to limit and regulate markets more efficiently. The purpose of this delineation and regulation would be to allow other spheres of activity and civil society to be conducted on non-economic lines. Thus they would be liberated from 'the colonisation of the lifeworld' whereby economic rationality and market values aided by the state bureaucracy come to subsume civil society (Gorz 1989a, 1993; Habermas 1987).

Post-industrial socialism is, then, a recipe for reducing the role of work in market settings and freeing up time for individuals to spend either working for themselves or their communities and engaging in self-determined activities. In this sense it is about emancipating communities, institutions of civil society and individuals rather than liberalising markets to pervade spheres of life where their influence may be detrimental. The post-industrial Left accepts a role for markets without surrendering socialist principles and imperatives, which is not the case with either market socialism or the social market economy. Unlike the latter two perspectives it definitively requires radical social and economic policies and this makes it more distant on the horizon. Nevertheless, it does provide a model of 'socialism with markets' which can act as a useful starting point in the debates which are likely to continue as socialism searches for a new agenda which will adequately combat the excesses and the unequal outcomes generated by the new economy.

Post-Fordism and post-industrialism

The latter part of this chapter is concerned with outlining the differences between post-industrial socialism and other concepts which have emerged in recent times, such as post-Fordism and post-modernity. The emergence of this new breed of 'postism' signals that qualitative changes have occurred in the organisation of advanced capitalism, although there is little agreement within the trend about what these changes actually entail. There is a common tendency within 'postism' to reject theoretical meta-narratives and utopian grand theorising about the 'good society' in the interests of a more pragmatic politics (although, of course, it is ironic that much post-modern discourse can be viewed as distinctly grand theory). The idea of the 'good society' remains central to post-industrial socialism, however, because, just as it rejects the technological determinism of most post-industrialist theorising, so it also operates on the level of theorising policies which could lead to a post-capitalist, post-materialist, non-work-based society. As we shall see below, socialist post-industrialism is opposed to the nihilistic bent of post-modernism. So while Pepper is correct in suggesting that a commitment to socialism should entail a rejection of the 'capitalist utopia' which results from conservative post-industrialism and post-modernism, he is incorrect in stating that 'postmodernism accompanies post-industrial theory' (Pepper 1993: 138). In other words, we can reject the opposition to universalist social theories inherent in post-modernism without surrendering the idea that a radical post-industrial society might be effective in achieving traditional socialist objectives. In this sense post-industrial socialism also rejects the attempts of commentators such as Leadbetter who pronounce that the viability of socialist politics is dependent on an interaction of post-modernism and post-Fordism which entails surrendering old ideas of 'rationality, order, power, authority, hierarchy and justice. Both attack that "one-big-narrative"' (Leadbetter 1989: 410). Rather, post-industrial socialists take the viewpoint that there is a necessity 'for modernity *itself to be modernised*, to be included reflexively in its own sphere of action: for *rationality itself to be rationalised*' (Gorz 1989a: 1; see also Beck 1992: 216-17).

The critique of post-Fordism

Post-Fordism differs from post-industrial socialism in the sense that the former is primarily concerned with analysing a phase of advanced capitalism while the latter is concerned with ways to create an alternative to contemporary capitalism. Theorists of post-Fordism tend to concentrate on changes in the world of work although some have attempted to outline broader ways in which post-Fordism becomes a force in culture and society (Hall and Jacques 1989). The debate has broadened in the 1990s with increasing contributions from political geographers and analyses of the implications of post-Fordism for the welfare state (for example Amin 1994b; Burrows and Loader 1994).[7] However, despite the generation of much discourse on post-Fordism, there has been little agreement about whether we have entered into a post-Fordist era.

As with industrialism and post-industrialism, the idea of post-Fordism is closely tied up with what it is supposed to have replaced, namely Fordism, which is linked to the application of the Taylorist division of labour by Henry Ford. The name suggests that, while numerous changes may have been made in the process of replacing one regime with another, some features of the old regime may still remain. Ritzer's definition suggests that there are five main features of Fordism: mass production of homogeneous goods; inflexible technological forms of production such as the assembly line; standardised Taylorist work routines; economies of scale, deskilling, intensification and homogeneous, interchangeable workers; and homogenised mass consumption to meet the growth of mass production (Ritzer 1993: 153–4). From an anti-deterministic perspective, it can be argued that the last point is the most vital if we are to judge whether societies as well as economies are Fordist or post-Fordist. In other words, the success or failure of Fordism was reliant on the ability to manufacture demand for the products which were being mass produced. Thus the success of the labour process model becomes reliant on the ability to generate conformity from those who are supposed to provide demand for the products which are being developed. In this sense, as Lipietz has suggested, the labour process model and the regime of accumulation require 'a mode of regulation' which 'involves all the mechanisms which adjust the contradictory and conflictual behaviour of individuals to the collective principles of the [macro-economic] regime of accumulation' (Lipietz 1993: 2).

Understood in this sense, there is broad, though not unanimous, agreement that the post-war era can be characterised as being Fordist and that that Fordism broke down in the period between the end of the 1960s and early 1970s. The post-war period is characterised by Lipietz as 'the golden age of Fordism', which mirrors other attempts to mark this era as 'the Keynesian consensus' or a 'welfare capitalist consensus' (Lipietz 1993: 14–23). While it would be wrong to suggest that there was no concurrence of mainstream political ideas in this period, the notions of the golden age and the consensus are a little misleading in terms of the variety of thought which existed beyond the pale of mainstream politics. They can obscure the amount of work devoted to demonstrating the failures of the 'golden age of consensus' such as that centred on the problems of Fordism and Taylorism (Gorz 1967) or the varied types of welfare capitalism which emerged in the post-war era (Esping-Andersen 1990). Nevertheless, it is fair to say that many of the principles of Fordist organisation were adopted in this era but also that Fordism was interdependent with Keynesian economic management and some form of Keynesian welfare state in producing an appropriate mode of regulation in which welfare capitalism could operate effectively in developed nations (Pierson 1995: 43–4). There can be little doubt now that the old system did break down in most of those countries, not least through governmental decisions that the system needed to be replaced. But what emerged after the fall of Fordism as a social and economic system?

Undoubtedly much has changed in the interim period but there is little agreement as to what format the changes have followed. Turning again to Ritzer, he suggests that the notion of Fordism being replaced by post-Fordism is premised upon five main assumptions: a qualitative change in the nature of consumption which has rendered mass production obsolete; specialised production which undermines economies of scale; the advent of flexibility enhanced by new technology; a reskilling of workers; and the birth of a new differentiated consumer (Ritzer 1993: 154–5). Few commentators take this to the extreme and contend that there has been a wholesale change in the organisation of Western societies (let alone the rest of the world) but Hall and Jacques, in their contribution to the post-Fordist debate in *New Times*, do go as far as to say 'post-Fordism is at the leading edge of change, increasingly setting the tone of society and providing the dominant rhythm of cultural change' (Hall and Jacques 1989: 12). Although most of the *New Times* contributors are careful not to ascribe deterministic economic power to changes in the labour market (Hall 1989: 119), that is precisely what they have been criticised for doing (Hirst 1989: 322). Hirst, like Hall, points to new developments in the labour process which he, along with many others, terms 'flexible specialisation' (see also Amin 1994a; Sabel 1994). According to Lash and Urry, 'the move from Taylorism and Fordism to flexibilization is an integral part of the disorganization of contemporary capitalist societies' (Lash and Urry 1987: 283). There appears to be agreement on the move towards flexible specialisation but that does not mean that we have entered into a post-Fordist era which offers radical new potentialities for the Left as is implied occasionally in *New Times*. Rather, the move towards flexible working must be recognised as an economic and political development which has occurred because it offers further scope for capitalist accumulation and reproduction. For post-industrial socialists, the massive growth of flexible labour patterns signifies a further step in the disintegration of social cohesion (Little 1997). Post-Fordist working patterns have hardened divisions between those in secure, well-paid work and those who become victims of the new flexibility because it spawns a wealth of peripheral, short-term employment. Moreover, as we shall see later, institutions such as the welfare state have not moved with the 'New Times', making it difficult to regulate conformity from those who are marginalised. This is precisely the reason why changes in the economy need to be met by the kinds of social policies which are evaluated towards the end of this book.

It seems that the notion of flexible specialisation has more utility for post-industrial socialists than post-Fordism because the former is more grounded in the notion of new forms of capitalist reproduction than the latter. Advocates of the Leftist potential of 'post-Fordist' developments have faced stern criticism for imputing too much qualitative change to what has become, in effect, a state of flux. Some elements of Fordism have broken down but many still remain within both Western capitalist economies and developing nations. Thus Ritzer states that 'elements of post-Fordism have emerged in the modern world, and yet it is equally clear that elements of Fordism persist and show no signs of disappearing' (Ritzer 1993: 155). For him, homogeneity, standardisation, rigid technologies and deskilled working are still rife in the global economy which he characterises as undergoing a phase of McDonaldisation. It appears, then, that post-Fordism is as culpable as conservative post-industrialism in engaging in premature 'postism'. This reinforces the post-industrial socialist viewpoint that post-industrial society (in the form of the end of work-based society) is something to be achieved rather than something which has emerged and is determining social relations.

Undoubtedly, post-Fordism can be a valuable concept in examining the growth of flexible specialisation in labour markets and the new economy but it should be approached with caution in regard to wider social organisation. It does not offer positive prospects for post-industrial socialists because it is firmly ingrained in and inexplicably linked with the contemporary mode of capitalist regulation. Thus it seems that, rather than accommodating Leftist potential, the changes associated with post-Fordism have been part of a complex recipe which has facilitated the growth of liberalised market policies throughout advanced capitalism, although the specific modes of regulation have varied (Esping-Andersen 1990). Post-industrial socialism, on the other hand, is being formulated around planning routes out of contemporary capitalism which entail reduced working hours for everyone in the economy and, interdependent with economic policy, more effective redistributive social policy based upon universalist principles.

Post-industrial socialism: a modern project?

In recent times many commentators have been moved to suggest the end of modernity and the beginning of a new post-modern era. For instance, Bauman claims that: 'With communism, the ghost of modernity has been exorcised' (Bauman 1992: 180). Post-industrial socialism, on the other hand, unlike other versions of 'postism', is a project consistent with the guiding principles of modernity. Unlike some defenders of post-Fordism, for instance, it makes no overtures to post-modernism (Leadbetter 1989). It perceives the world as being rationally intelligible even if we cannot ensure strict knowledge of outcomes. Post-industrial socialism has at its root the primacy of values such as mutualism, co-operation, equality, solidarity, inclusion, community and cohesiveness, and attempts to identify policy issues which could lead to a society which embraces those values. The most renowned proponent of post-industrial socialism, André Gorz, is notable for grand, utopian theory and meta-narratives (Gorz 1982; see also Geoghegan 1987). Indeed, Gorz is explicitly concerned with reflexivity which Giddens claims is intrinsic to (late or high) modernity and Beck's 'new modernist' notion of 'risk society' (Giddens 1991: 19–21, 28).[8] Obviously, any attempt to formulate an end to work-based society by initiating policies that are made possible by current conditions is likely to be anathema to post-modernists. Gorz's perspective on modernity and rationality is exemplified by the following passage:

> What we are experiencing is not the crisis of modernity. We are experiencing the need to modernize the presuppositions upon which modernity is based. The current crisis is not the crisis of Reason but that of (increasingly apparent) irrational motives of rationalization as it has been pursued thus far . . . What 'post-modernists' take to be the end of modernity and the crisis of Reason is in reality the crisis of the quasi-religious irrational contents upon which the selective and partial rationalization we call industrialism – bearer of a conception of the universe and a vision of the future which are now untenable – is based.
>
> (Gorz 1989a: 1)

In other words, Gorz suggests that we have not been catapulted into a post-modern age by a crisis of modernist rationality – the crisis that exists is one where what is seen to be rational has stagnated within the confines of existing industrialism. In this sense post-industrialism (as Gorz understands it) is a modernist project which has been hindered by the hegemony of economic rationality. This economic rationality is the key component of market-based industrial society which has run out of steam, according to Gorz. He claims that the project of modernity can only be continued by transcending the stranglehold of capitalist industrialism underpinned by economic rationality and formulating a coherent socialist post-industrial agenda. In this sense the reaction to the crisis of industrialism should not be the abandonment of rational concepts of modernity as is the case with post-modernism, rather it should be the restatement of modernist goals within a post-industrial framework. Thus it is the inability to see beyond the artificially imposed boundaries of industrialism which has left space for post-modernists to assert the crisis of modernity. Gorz notes that 'as long as we remain bound by this vision, we will continue to cling to individual pursuits and nostalgic views of the past, incapable of giving either meaning or direction to the changes which have caused the destruction of our past beliefs' (Gorz 1989a: 1).

A similar point is made by Wagner, even though he approaches the question from a different angle from that of Gorz. The former notes that roles, identities and institutions of modernity, such as those related to labour and unemployment, had to be created and as such the reconstitution of society and the role of work therein is clearly a modernist project. Wagner rejects the post-modernist critique of modernity as an 'inverse fallacy' in which 'postmodernists rather fail to provide the needed critique of modernity' (Wagner 1994: 23). Just as Gorz invites a critique of modernity in terms of industrialism, so Wagner also recognises that modernity requires thorough analysis which has not been a feature of much post-modernist work which is *ad hominem* in its critique. Positing a new era in a traditional 'postist' fashion is no substitute for critical evaluation. The crisis of modernity, insofar as it can be said to exist, appears to be the inability to analyse modernity while still recognising that the answer may still lie within modernity itself. For Gorz, the answer within modernity is to think the unthinkable and dare to envisage policies leading to a post-industrial order equipped with appropriate socialist values. This fits in with Beck's analysis of 'risk society' where he reasons that: '*Just as modernization dissolved the structure of feudal society in the nineteenth century and produced the industrial society, modernization today is dissolving industrial society and another modernity is coming into being*' (Beck 1992: 10). Thus a new modernity may be forming which is characterised by a fusion of features of both the old political relations of modernity and newer features associated with post-modernity (perhaps in the cultural sphere).[9] Indeed, in what follows in the rest of this book an attempt will be made to outline potential models for post-industrial welfare which, it could be argued, have benefited from the growth of post-modernism and the accompanying celebration of diversity and divergence (Williams 1994). This is not to say, of course, that a post-modern theory of welfare will be presented (Leonard 1997). On the contrary, the models examined are regarded as being part of a process within the new modernity: namely, socialist post-industrialism.

Conclusion

This chapter has attempted to provide a background framework for the idea of post-industrial socialism in the light of the main competing theoretical perspectives. It is to all extents and purposes a political framework for change rather than a purely descriptive label for changes in labour markets or broader cultural changes. The post-industrial socialist approach rejects the economic determinism of some forms of post-Fordism and the uninitiated adoption of 'the market' by market socialists and social market theorists. Rather, it attempts to outline a model for 'socialism with markets' which recognises that the labour process must be highly regulated and subjected in importance to activities which are not concerned necessarily with 'work for wages'. This is presented as a process which is profoundly modernist in the sense that it is concerned with the creation of a new post-industrial modernity. In this sense post-industrial socialism is grounded in the production of the future from the realities of living in the present and, as such, it must be regarded as inimical to post-modernism. Most importantly, though, this is primarily a socialist programme which in this book will focus on the politics of work and welfare. It should not be equated with the kind of post-industrialism which was heralded by Bell in the 1970s or that which is accepted as existing by Esping-Andersen and Clement and Myles. This book is intended as a contribution to ongoing debates on the future of social policy in Europe. It is neither a prediction nor a tentative exercise in futurology but rather an attempt to apply new ideas in social and political theory to contemporary directions in welfare theory.

2

THE POST-INDUSTRIAL
SOCIALIST CRITIQUE OF THE
WELFARE STATE

Post-industrial socialism has emanated mainly from Western Europe and it is clearly concerned with presenting a viable alternative to welfare capitalism. This is not to say that the values underpinning post-industrial socialism are not equally applicable in other parts of the world but rather that, in the search to find routes to a more equitable future from present conditions, post-industrial socialists tend to focus on the state of advanced capitalist societies and the potential for change therein. One of the central features of Left-libertarian theory is the critique of the welfare state and the outline of potential socialist alternatives for post-industrial social policy. The post-industrial socialist critique of the welfare state owes much to the perspectives of neo-Marxism, feminism and political ecology, although it also accepts some of the elements of the neo-liberal critique of the welfare state without sharing the political sentiment underpinning the latter. Initially this chapter will focus on the areas of convergence and divergence between the neo-Marxist and neo-liberal approaches to the welfare state before moving on to highlight the features of feminist and anti-racist critiques which have also informed the post-industrial socialist perspective. The concluding section will highlight the main principles of the latter and the similarities with and differences from the angle of political ecology. To begin with, though, it is appropriate to analyse briefly some of the key social democratic ideas and principles related to the Keynesian welfare state (KWS) and the state of social welfare in general.

There is a wealth of literature on the development of the Keynesian welfare state and the historical factors which heralded the development of Western European welfare capitalism.[1] The main focus here will be on the economic and social factors which underpinned the KWS and the different factors which have undermined the foundations of welfare capitalism. The KWS was founded on the basis of two main interdependent principles. First, there would be 'macro-management of the economy to ensure economic growth under conditions of full employment' (Pierson 1991: 28) and, second, there would be state provision of a range of social services which would help to redistribute resources to those in need of them. The successful achievement of the former would provide sufficient resources to implement the latter and the number of people in need would be limited in any case because of full (male) employment. In this sense the KWS was fundamentally reliant on favourable economic conditions prevailing. This is borne out by the fact that Keynes himself rarely had much to say about social welfare, as well as the idea that his effect on social policy was indirect and due mainly to his preoccupation with unemployment (Williams and Williams 1995: 73, 76). Thus the development (and affordability) of the KWS was closely linked with the eradication of unemployment which necessitated a range of measures including policies designed to maintain traditional gender roles in the post-war reconstruction and the widespread implementation of Fordism in the economy. Indeed, Jessop suggests that 'if the Keynesian welfare state helped to secure the conditions for Fordist economic expansion, the latter helped in turn to secure the conditions for the expansion of the Keynesian welfare state' (Jessop 1994a: 256). As we saw in the last chapter, there is widespread agreement that Fordism, as the central component of economic organisation, has broken down. If this is the case, following Jessop (although not necessarily going along with his conception of post-Fordism), it seems pertinent to note that the demise of Fordism destroyed one of the key dimensions of the KWS. What is at issue, then, is whether the waning of Keynesian economic arrangements has signalled a terminal crisis for the welfare state.

Literature on the crisis of the welfare state poured forth from both neo-liberals and neo-Marxists from the 1970s onwards (Hill 1993; Hindess 1987; Klein 1993). The post-industrial socialist approach to welfare takes on board many of the sentiments of crisis literature without suggesting that the welfare state and/or the economic system stand on the precipice of apocalyptic collapse. Rather, it notes crisis tendencies and seeks to examine transitional movements in which either advanced capitalist societies instigate policies to assure their reproduction or where openings may occur for socialist policies to develop. From the perspective of post-industrial socialism the welfare state has alleviated some social problems and accentuated others. As such it cannot necessarily be regarded as an egalitarian institution because, as Baker suggests, 'the present welfare state is a compromise which serves many interests. It helps people in need, but it also helps to keep them in their place. It is a system of support but also of control.' In short, Baker argues that 'the welfare state is designed for an unequal society' (Baker 1987: 10). The post-industrial socialist approach to social welfare is premised upon what Clarke calls 'deep citizenship' which entails 'personal identity and integrity, autonomy, mutuality and social and political responsibility'. This necessitates 'a significant pro-active educational and welfare commitment. Such a commitment is not to be regretted as a drain on society. It is rather to be welcomed as an opportunity by which society can lift itself to new heights' (Clarke 1996: 114–15).

A welfare crisis: neo-liberalism and neo-Marxism

Initially it is important to note that, although there is great diversity in sentiment both within and between the two ideological standpoints, there appear to be several areas of convergence in the critiques of the welfare state developed by neo-liberals and neo-Marxists (Kenny and Little 1995: 285; Stoesz and Midgley 1991: 30). Both perspectives subscribed to the crisis of the welfare state thesis in the 1970s and 1980s, although they did so for very different reasons. Neo-liberals pointed to the crisis as an example of the inefficiency of state intervention in the economy and the poverty of Keynesian economic management. This enabled 'neo-liberalism . . . to launch an all-out ideological offensive under the themes of "the bankruptcy of socialism" and "market capitalism – the response to the crisis"' (Gorz 1985: 7). Neo-Marxists, on the other hand, were more concerned with criticising post-war social democratic governments who used the KWS to present a humane face of capitalism while failing to deal with the problems that the KWS actually created. Thus Offe states that 'the Keynesian welfare state is a "victim of its success" . . . the side effects of its successful practice of solving *one* type of macro-economic problem have led to the emergence of an *entirely different problematique*, one which is beyond the steering capacity of the KWS' (Offe 1984: 200). Clearly, there is some concurrence on the failings of Keynesianism but there is little agreement on alternatives to the KWS. While neo-Marxists have continued their critical analysis of trends in state welfare by moving on to, for example, Offe's 'non-productivist design for social policies' (Offe 1992), neo-liberals have had more success in actually influencing governmental ideology, especially in the United Kingdom and the USA in the 1980s and 1990s, although public expenditure as a percentage of GDP actually rose in both countries between 1970 and 1990 (George and Page 1995a: 10).[2]

The natural order and the economy: the
neo-liberal approach

The two key figures in developing neo-liberal theories of social policy are the Nobel Prize-winning monetarist economists, F. A. Hayek and Milton Friedman.[3] Just as was the case with his opponent, Keynes, Hayek's influence on social policy debates was somewhat tangential and his main focus was on the infringements of individual liberty that occurred as a result of state planning and economic management (Hayek 1991; Tomlinson 1995: 21). Friedman, on the other hand, has been more explicit about the relationship between his philosophy of economic emancipation and social welfare policies (Friedman 1982: 177–89). The central thrust with both writers, though, is the liberalisation of the economy from state intervention which would lead to a spontaneous natural social order (catallaxy) in Hayek's view (Pierson 1991: 42; Hindess 1987: 127–8) or, for Friedman, an opportunity for freedom to flourish safe from the threat of 'concentration of power' (Friedman 1982: 2). Clearly, both Hayek and Friedman are more concerned with the economy, freedom of 'the market' and individual (negative) liberty than social welfare.[4] What emerges from their work, then, is an idea of how individual welfare would improve with an unfettered market rather than a coherent theory of social welfare itself. Welfare, it is assumed, is generated by free individuals engaging in activity in 'the market' with a very limited safety net for the very worst off who do not or cannot survive in the market place. Pierson notes that 'this last duty to relieve destitution is not to be identified with the welfare state. Relief is not a statutory right of citizenship, but needs-based and discretionary' (Pierson 1991: 44).

The opposition to the welfare state in Friedman's case is built upon an antipathy to mandatory contributions to public institutional monopolies, graduated income taxes and government subsidisation of welfare programmes. Not only does he object to the methods of funding welfare provision but he also makes a point that is central to the neo-liberal critique: namely, that state provision has been wholly ineffective in delivering the services that it is supposed to. In *Capitalism and Freedom* he uses the example of public housing programmes to show that state intervention had not significantly improved the housing conditions of the poor. Friedman suggests that it would be better to replace assistance programmes with cash benefits:

> [T]he families being helped would rather have a given sum in cash than in the form of housing. They could themselves spend the money on housing if they so desired. Hence, they would

> never be worse off if given cash; if they regarded other needs as
> more important, they would be better off.
>
> (Friedman 1982: 178)

This is symptomatic of the kind of pecuniary approach to solving dilemmas of social welfare that neo-liberals tend to favour. Friedman assumes that the welfare of individuals and society can be assured so long as they have or are given sums of money regardless of the various ills that capitalist society may engender. He believes that as long as people have economic power to purchase and consume products, then they are 'free to choose' which voluntary exchanges they take part in, regulated by the price mechanism. Quite rightly Hindess takes Friedman to task for ignoring 'institutional circumstances' such as the prior distribution of resources before voluntary exchanges. In the end this comes down to chance. Hindess asserts that Friedman's 'simplistic' social analysis 'reduces to three interacting elements: human individuals making choices, governments interfering, and chance' (Hindess 1987: 126). Even more sympathetic commentators to neo-liberal ideas such as Barry observe that:

> Friedman's account of liberty is perhaps not too sophisticated. It
> consists of a somewhat crude version of 'negative' liberty: that is,
> the idea that a person is free to the extent that his or her actions
> are not restrained by coercive law. He shows little interest in
> enquiring into the social and economic conditions that may
> make one person's freedom more valuable than another's, or
> into sources of constraint on human action other than law and
> politics; and least of all in considering the possibility that col-
> lectively supplied welfare might increase people's autonomy or
> their sense of citizenship.
>
> (Barry 1995: 34)

This latter point is significant in terms of formulating social policies along Friedmanite lines. There is little attempt in his work to outline concrete social relations and methods through which individuals would unite, co-operate and bind as citizens. The only domain in which co-operation genuinely enters Friedman's equation is in market transactions, reinforcing the idea that Friedman subverts all else to economics. In any case his discussion of voluntary transactions seriously distorts the nature of relations in markets and sanitises market relationships from any form of exploitation. His glorification of 'the market' is clearly at odds with the thinking of post-industrial socialism not least because he makes

41

no attempt to suggest ways in which the state may be able to offset the inadequacies and pitfalls of markets. Thus the essential aim of Friedmanite conservatives is 'not of eradicating poverty and unemployment, but of making them socially acceptable at the least cost to society. Dualistic social stratification is therefore inevitably maintained, and even reinforced' (Gorz 1985: 41).

There are some areas, however, where the work of neo-liberals such as Friedman and Hayek can find currency in socialist debates: namely, the inadequacy of the welfare state in efficiently providing security, solidarity and citizenship, and the importance of economics to social policy debates. This does not mean that neo-liberals are justified in outlining an extremely limited role for the state in the economy and social welfare but rather acknowledges that the welfare state has not been developed sufficiently in recent times to move with the new economy. As mentioned in Chapter 1, the post-industrial socialist perspective relies on state planning to regulate the parameters of market relations which is anathema to the Hayekian critique of the state which is based upon the belief that 'planning cannot replicate the orderly mutual adjustment of the market because it can never marshal all the required knowledge in one place' (Hindess 1987: 128). This may well be the case but Hayek assumes that we cannot know outcomes in a market-based society as if there were no alternative to that kind of society. Post-industrial socialism does not aim to abolish markets; the target is market-based society. By minimising the sphere of markets, they can be more easily regulated and subject to planning. Even Hayek, as inveterate a defender of 'the market' as anyone (but in a rather contradictory way at times), goes as far as to say 'it is impossible to direct industry without exercising some influence on distribution' in the middle of a passage which claims that planning in an economy will lead to comprehensive planning throughout the economy (Hayek 1991: 79).[5] Clearly, post-industrial socialism can learn a little from neo-liberalism in terms of criticising the effectiveness of the welfare state but ultimately there is nothing within the latter perspective which holds potential for the maximisation of social welfare – the primary area of investigation of this book. A more fruitful ground for realising this aim may lie within the neo-Marxist analysis of the welfare state.

Contradictions and the return of the crisis: neo-Marxist analysis

The neo-Marxist crisis perspective which emerged in the 1970s and 1980s is most commonly associated with the work of Ian Gough (1979), James O'Connor (1973, 1984) and Claus Offe (1984, 1985). Both Gough and

O'Connor favoured the notion of fiscal crisis, whereby the state could no longer perform the contradictory role of maximising capital accumulation and ensuring political legitimacy. Offe, on the other hand, sees a crisis of crisis management, whereby the primary role of the state is to manage the type of crisis that Gough and O'Connor recognise. For Offe, this crisis management throws up new contradictions which generate a new crisis of the state. It is this latter approach, one which views crisis tendencies as part of a process rather than as catastrophic events, which is favoured here (Offe 1984: 36–7). In the 1990s a tendency has developed which treats the neo-Marxist critics of the welfare state as Jeremiahs who were prematurely heralding the demise of welfare capitalism (Klein 1993; Hill 1993; see also Lindblom 1996). Since the middle of the 1980s there has been a decline in crisis literature and many commentators are beginning to treat this period of crisis theory as a historical phase in the progress of the welfare state which has now been successfully overcome. Mishra, for example, divides the 'recent history of the welfare state' into three phases: 'pre-crisis (before 1973), crisis (the mid–late 1970s), and post-crisis (the 1980s and beyond)' (Mishra 1990: xii) without recourse to the notion that crises can occur and recur and be overcome without *crisis tendencies* being removed. Similarly, Klein makes a 'simple observation' that 'the welfare state in capitalist societies has survived the crisis in remarkably good health' (Klein 1993: 7). This is indeed a simple observation for it does not do justice to the work that Klein criticises.[6] Offe, in particular, is well aware that crisis tendencies can exist in welfare capitalist societies without necessarily bringing them to the brink of destruction. Kellner states that:

> Offe proposes that we abandon both the notion of a final crisis –
> that is, that a system-ending apocalypse is on the horizon – and
> the assumption that the system has produced techniques and
> strategies to manage the system indefinitely, and adopt instead
> a notion of 'the crisis of crisis management'.
>
> (Kellner 1989: 201)

Indeed, from the post-industrial socialist perspective, the reproduction of capitalism is likely to generate new and different crises which the system must overcome in some way to continue reproduction. It is only by highlighting areas of crisis and contradiction that the Left may be able to take advantage and attempt to implement change. In other words, it is the *job* of the post-industrial Left to identify crises in the capitalist system – but this does not mean that systemic collapse is imminent. The post-industrial Left, then, faces an unpopular task of continuing to examine developments in politics, society and the economy in order to delineate avenues for change. That task is not appreciated by the likes of Klein, who believes that: 'Diagnosing "contradictions", i.e. conflicts, in societies does not get us very far' (Klein 1993: 16). He should bear in mind that social and political change is often not brought about by sudden collapse but by conflicts existing over substantial periods of time. The post-industrial Left would be reneging on its duty if it did not continue to highlight crises in the nature of the capitalist system even if the chances of change look bleak. This is a more daunting task than that of commentators such as Klein who, comforted by 'the end of the crisis', wish away any need for change.

There is much that a post-industrial Left can learn from the neo-Marxist analyses of crises of the 1970s and early 1980s, not least the ways in which welfare capitalist societies and their welfare states have proved to be resilient against the problems which they have faced. Moreover, there is much to be gained from evaluating the inability of the Left to capitalise upon the crises which welfare capitalism faced in the 1970s in terms of providing systematic theoretical alternatives. The Left would also do well to recognise that crises would probably emerge in a different socialist society and that the complex nature of socio-economic arrangements will entail fluctuating political debates over appropriate policies (Dunleavy and O'Leary 1987: 266). For our purposes we shall focus on what the post-industrial socialist project has to learn from the work of Offe as his recent work has a close resonance with the idea of moving beyond the work-based society.[7] In recent times Offe has made some extremely useful contributions to the development of post-industrial socialist thought (Offe 1992; Offe and Heinze 1992). He has moved beyond his earlier work on the declining political support for the welfare state in attempting to outline a sphere of debate in which radical alternatives for state welfare could be developed which could generate widespread support. This project is based upon a rejection of European social democratic welfare strategies which are premised upon the rights and duties of employees rather than citizens (Offe 1992: 70). The main thrust, which sits comfortably with the work of Gorz and of Keane (1988), for example, is the limitation of state power and the regeneration of democratic civil society.[8] This provides an opportunity for dialogue between the post-industrial Left and other ideological traditions such as feminism and political ecology which have challenged orthodox notions about activity in the private and public spheres and the statist and industrialist nature of many theoretical debates about welfare (Ferris 1985: 71).

It is evident that Offe has not moved away from his early neo-Marxist notions of contradictions of the welfare state and the crisis of crisis management as he maintains that a 'persistent issue in the ongoing social and political conflict over the operational meaning of social security and welfare concerns the supply side – the fiscal resources that are necessary to cover recognized needs' (Offe 1992: 63). This refutes Dean's claim that Offe's more recent work (particularly that co-written with Heinze, 1992) is 'especially remote from the neo-Marxist theoretical tradition' (Dean 1995: 232). This is symptomatic of the reception received by post-Marxist policy proposals which are designed to envisage an alternative to contemporary capitalism. The boundary between acceptable analysis of welfare capitalism and the 'utopian' process of setting out alternative futures for the Left is exceptionally stringent for most commentators. Offe's more recent work on basic income and the nature of work is a clear extension of his earlier analyses of the labour market in *Disorganized Capitalism* (1985), for example. It is only from his neo-Marxist theoretical basis that he is able to move on to proposals for non-productivist social policies. Most of the theorists associated with the post-industrial Left have been unfairly castigated for presenting alternative 'utopian' strategies to the present. This seems to be extremely retrograde for the Left in general as it will be toothless in the face of resilient capitalism if it is unable even to countenance the messy task of imagining the future (Little 1996: ch. 8; Geoghegan 1987).

Offe is keen to refute the productivist logic which is a key foundation of welfare capitalist welfare states. Thus he reasons that 'they are centred on the notion that production and productivity are both individually and collectively desirable, and hence on the morally self-evident criterion of material reward' (Offe 1992: 67). This productivist base for the welfare state is, according to Offe, increasingly discordant with the realities of disorganised capitalism because the assumptions productivist social policy embraces are increasingly incongruous with everyday life. Offe lists five of these assumptions. First, the productivist welfare state was reliant upon the existence of families which performed an important 'micro' social security network for family members. Second, each family would have at least one breadwinner to provide a family wage and thereby reduce the necessity for recourse to welfare. Third, conflicts over the system of distribution would be negotiated and legitimated by a range of collective actors. Fourth, the welfare state would exist to resolve any problems that were not satisfied by either families or representative collective actors. Finally, the welfare state (and the funds extracted from citizens to pay for it) would be relatively uncontroversial as there would be a general consensus because citizens would realise the benefits (e.g. health care) that they derived from it. For Offe, 'these . . . assumptions have become much harder to accept as valid and reliable representations of the social and economic reality of advanced industrial societies . . .

[they] are undergoing symptoms of stress and widely perceived insecurity' (Offe 1992: 68–9).

This scenario is a useful summary of some of the main elements of the post-industrial socialist critique of the welfare state. From this it is clear that the problems of the welfare state go beyond political economy. While elements of a fiscal crisis may still remain and may well get worse as demographic changes occur and the availability of sufficient work declines, the problems of the welfare state go much deeper. This approach is founded in the idea that the social institutions which underpinned the development of welfare states have changed in a variety of ways, thereby shaking the foundations of the welfare state as we know it. Thus arrangements for state welfare have lacked flexibility and the state has proved inept at transforming welfare provision to suit new social and economic conditions. Increasingly the political legitimacy of the welfare state is weakened by the demise of the nuclear family, the new flexibility in labour markets, the increasing lack of influence on the political process for individuals and collective actors, and the heavy demand placed on the welfare state due to the above factors. In this situation there is decreasing consensus about the format of state welfare accompanied by increased social division and disintegration. In other words, state welfare is being attacked from many directions but, at the same time, social welfare is also deteriorating. The key for post-industrial socialists is to regenerate state welfare and social consensus about what form that welfare provision should take, against the hegemony of neo-liberal thought which effectively severs state responsibility from social welfare. Before clarifying the post-industrial socialist critique of the welfare state, it is necessary to examine elements of the feminist and anti-racist critiques of the welfare state which have informed the perspective of the post-industrial Left.

Feminism and anti-racism[9]

As with any other ideological perspectives, there are wide varieties within feminism and anti-racism, so the features attributed to the critiques here should not be regarded as prescriptive to all standpoints within the two traditions.[10] This account, then, will examine elements within feminism and anti-racism, rather than attempt to provide a definitive statement of what each perspective entails. In terms of the changing nature of work and welfare, the traditional concern with difference and diversity that have characterised feminism and anti-racism are of central importance to post-industrial socialism. Essentially we 'need to take account not only of the changing conditions of work but of the changing conditions of family, culture and nationhood too, and that these should be understood in terms of the changing relations not only of class, but of other social divisions, including gender and "race"' (Williams 1994: 72).

The politics of difference and universalism: feminist approaches

George and Wilding highlight a number of key points which are relevant to the feminist analysis of welfare. They note that feminists (like postindustrial socialists) are generally ambivalent towards the welfare state primarily because it does not recognise the particularity of women's needs and serves to reinforce traditional gender roles. Moreover, feminists argue against the welfare state because it fails to engage with the vital relations within the private sphere; it is set up according to male-dominated value systems; it provides low-paid, part-time employment which is mainly populated by women; and, lastly, it is sexist at root because policymaking procedures are dominated by men (George and Wilding 1994: 137–49). These issues have been moved to the centre of social policy debates by feminist writers. Thus Williams states that 'in demanding a changed basis to the relationship between the welfare state and women, feminists have . . . made the issues of *who* controls welfare and how it is organised . . . questions of immediate concern and political priority' (Williams 1989: 86). Towards the end of this book, we shall see that postindustrial socialism may have something to offer feminists in terms of the furtherance of their objectives in future social policy.

Given the centrality of work to post-industrial socialism, the issue of women and work is a point on which there is considerable convergence in thought with feminism. Indeed, most of the thinkers that can be linked with post-industrial socialism such as Offe and Gorz have engaged in a variety of debates about women and work. These theorists are quick to point to not only the position of women within the labour market, but also the vital issue of women and domestic labour. For instance, Offe notes that:

> The dependency of workers upon the particular job they have, with relatively inferior 'exit' options *in* the labour market, is most clearly evident in circumstances where a dual role is not merely a possibility that must be anticipated, but already a constituent element of the actual situation. The best and most well-known example is the actual double burdening of many women by occupational activity and domestic responsibilities. 'Working housewives' are typically deprived of some of their

capacity to adapt to market opportunities and can only deploy their labour power within narrow spatial and temporal limits.

(Offe 1985: 42)

Keane and Gorz concur with the thrust of Offe's argument by pointing to a 'double shift' whereby women undertake a substantial majority of domestic work and increasingly work in the public sphere as well for less remuneration, less security and frequently in poorer conditions with less organised representation. Gorz suggests that this situation is an outrage which is 'doubly iniquitous and doubly scandalous' (Gorz 1994: 92). From a feminist perspective, Williams also points to the fact that much female employment in the public sphere may replicate domestic activities in the home. This is particularly the case for women welfare workers such as 'cooks, cleaners, carers, educators and so on', although she also notes Carby's point that 'the racist image of *Black woman as servant* is as strong as that of *carer* in the acceptance of Black women in domestic, nursing and cleaning roles' (Williams 1989: 77; also see Pascall 1986: 50). It is clear that, while women have increasingly entered work in the public sphere since the early post-war years, they are entering a rather closed labour market which is divided and segregated along gender lines. Bryson (1992: 157) refers to this as a move from 'private patriarchy to public patriarchy'.

It should be clear from the above that post-industrial socialists share much of the feminist interpretation of women and work and that the former are presenting a socialist critique of work and welfare that goes beyond traditional socialist theories which focused on male, manual workers (Mishra 1984: 93). Of course, this can be taken too far, as is the case when Esping-Andersen uncritically heralds more work for women in the new 'post-industrial' era as opposed to the old traditional state of affairs:

> The revolutionary essence of the emerging post-industrial society lies very much in its abolition of . . . [the old] gender logic. First, as the realm of social services expands, the necessity of household self-reproduction declines, thus freeing women from traditional family care obligations . . . Service jobs are not only more flexible and less physically demanding, but they are also frequently 'natural' female career avenues in the sense that they offer paid employment in what are essentially traditional social reproduction tasks. Services for women create jobs for women.
>
> (Esping-Andersen 1993: 17)

Esping-Andersen's statement is inherently productivist, resting as it does on the old ethos that 'any job is better than no job'. The 'post-industrialism' that he celebrates does not necessarily abolish the old gender logic. If that were the case women would not be primarily employed in service jobs which are socially constructed as 'natural female career avenues' (Williams 1989: 181–2).[11] What's more, Esping-Andersen falls into the trap of assuming that, just because more women are employed in the public sphere, they necessarily do less work in the domestic sphere. While technological developments mean that women (and men) may spend less *time* doing domestic tasks, this does not mean that domestic labour is being shared equally by men and women. On the contrary, Tyrrell has recently provided evidence that this is patently not the case and that working women still perform much more work in the private sphere than men (Tyrrell 1995: 25). The 'post-industrial' logic that Esping-Andersen celebrates is only a sign that the process of moving towards a service economy (tertiarisation) has provided employment for women in the public sphere which does little more than replicate many of the tasks that women have traditionally performed in the private sphere. The fact that there is payment for these tasks in the former does not necessarily make it economically rational or particularly fulfilling for those that perform them. This is not to say that we should disregard the importance of the increasing entrance of women into the labour market in terms of access to the public sphere, but rather that we should question the type of work that the majority of women are segregated into in the tertiarised economy. Again the point that post-industrial socialism is vastly different from mainstream post-industrialism is self-evident in comparing the ideas of Esping-Andersen with those of Gorz, Keane or Offe. As Nixon and Williamson point out, 'a segregated workforce is an international phenomenon, with women concentrated both in a small number of industrial categories and in particular types of work' (Nixon and Williamson 1993: 113).[12] The issue, then, becomes a means of socialising the labour market to provide more equity in the types of work performed by men and women in both the public and private spheres. The goal becomes the achievement of a more coherent 'work portfolio' for *everyone* in which there is an appropriate balance of paid and unpaid work (Handy 1990).

Clearly, the interaction of feminism and post-industrial socialism is particularly convergent on the nature and future of work. However, the post-industrial Left also shares much of the feminist critique of the welfare state. Pierson makes the point that despite the failings of the welfare state with regards to women, feminists should seek the solutions to their qualms within state welfare rather than outside of it (Pierson 1991: 221).

This echoes the feelings of the post-industrial Left that while the welfare state deserves much criticism, the best hope for universal social welfare lies in state responsibility for provision (Gorz 1989a: 208). Feminists are correct to highlight the role of the state in reinforcing social relations (and indeed in isolating the state as an embodiment of patriarchy), but post-industrial socialists argue for a state that is democratically accountable to communities and institutions in civil society. Thus democratic accountability can only be opposed to patriarchy if the implementation of stronger social (and economic) rights of citizenship are designed in ways which would 'feminise' the state (Holmwood 1993: 115). This assumes that communities, for example, must not be regarded as morally authoritarian and exclusivist institutions, but rather as bodies in which mutual values, voluntarism and friendship prevail and which have equal prominence with relations between individuals and the state (Hughes and Little 1996). The potential values of community (understood in the broadest sense) outlined above have a strong resonance with many feminist objectives (Friedman 1992). Post-industrial socialists, then, have as an objective the reconstruction of state welfare which incorporates the main aspects of the feminist critique of the welfare state. This involves radical alterations to economic policy which will proactively seek to desegregate the labour market and improve the place of women therein. This process will go hand in hand with reforms of social policy designed to ensure equity for each individual citizen. The bottom line of this process is recognition of the equal (but different) value of activities carried out in the public and private spheres and to ensure a more equal distribution of both types of work between women and men (and indeed other categories of people who experience different types of marginalisation such as those with disabilities). In other words, the task becomes a process of highlighting 'emancipatory possibilities of the present and . . . [anticipating] the conditions of a non-repressive, egalitarian, post-capitalist, and post-patriarchal society of the future' (d'Entreves 1994: 63). The tentative proposals for achieving these objectives (partly, at least) will be outlined in detail in Chapters 5 and 6 of this book.

Diversity and particularism: anti-racist theories of welfare

In the desire to create a state welfare proposal which is anti-discriminatory, post-industrial socialism shares much with the anti-racist perspective as well as feminism.[13] Here the focus will be on creating policies which are universal, yet allow individuals and communities to satisfy their needs in particularistic methods. This is vital because, as with the feminist perspective, anti-racism is founded upon the notion that different ethnic groups have different, divergent needs which in turn may be satisfied in a variety of ways. The challenge for the post-industrial Left is to formulate a framework in which universal state social policy develops inclusive citizenship while not prescribing the ways in which people must behave in their communities. This involves a process of outlining the values and responsibilities inherent in cohesive communities and the state and the possibility of cultural pluralism based on an effective partnership between the two. For Parekh, 'encouraging cohesive communities to run their own affairs themselves under the overall authority of the state is an important dimension of that partnership' (Parekh 1994: 107). Thus 'anti-racism . . . is not merely a defensive ideology and strategy. It is also a positive, forward-looking approach for the creation of harmonious multiethnic societies' (George and Page 1995b: 312). Initially, however, it is important to highlight the failings of the welfare state as anti-racists see it. Pierson provides two core ideas which underpin the anti-racist critique of the welfare state concerning the position of ethnic groups:

> First, their economically and socially less privileged position tends to make them more reliant upon provision through the welfare state. Secondly, this welfare state upon which they are peculiarly dependent treats them on systematically less favourable terms than members of the majority community.
>
> (Pierson 1991: 80)

In this sense anti-racists see the welfare state as inherently discriminatory. It has firm roots in the notion of national citizenship which immediately assigns an identity of 'otherness' on immigrants, refugees, asylum seekers, and so on. Moreover, the rights of individuals and communities belonging to minority ethnic groups who are already resident citizens come to be tarred with the same brush. The fact that ethnic groups may be more reliant as a proportion of overall numbers on the welfare state than majority groups means that backlashes against public spending and discourses on 'welfare scroungers' become more focused on ethnic groups (Kitschelt 1995). As such, ethnic minorities became the target of what Hall has called the authoritarian populism of hegemonic right-wing government in the United Kingdom (Denney 1995: 315). Also anti-racists point to the fact that members of minority ethnic groups may have less accessibility to some welfare benefits than the majority population. Thus Pierson argues that 'some sort of residence qualification for relief is a commonplace of public welfare which long predates the coming of the welfare state' (Pierson 1991: 80; see also Williams 1989: 158). This is all the more worrying when we take into account the existent and growing trend of 'intertwining . . . immigration control and welfare agencies' (Williams 1989: 143). On top of these general points we should also note that there is a variety of more specific policy issues linked to discrimination against minority ethnic groups which range across the welfare state from ghettoisation as a result of housing policy to the underachievement of some ethnic groups in the education system.[14] All of these features of the anti-racist critique should become vital tenets of the post-industrial socialist programme for social policy, based as it is on the eradication of discriminatory practices and the establishment of solidarity. Thus 'the new ethnic minorities of Western Europe are a natural constituency of concern for a Left concerned with inequalities of power and opportunity. Racial equality and minority rights are issues which should be integral to a European politics of social justice' (Modood 1994: 87). The key area where post-industrial socialism interacts with these issues is the relationship between work and welfare and no account of anti-racism and the welfare state can ignore the significance of the work of minority ethnic groups.

Tariq Modood gives a useful summary of the historical roots of the work of minority ethnic groups:

> Post-war Europe needed cheap labour to perform unskilled and unwanted jobs in an expanding economy, and the bulk of the migrations occurred in response to this need. The new ethnic minorities therefore entered European society at the bottom. That situation has more or less persisted for four decades. While some groups have an educational and economic profile similar to or perhaps better then the average of the European country in question . . . on the whole migrants and their descendants suffer much higher levels of unemployment than white people . . . The majority of those in employment are in unskilled and semi-skilled work.
>
> (Modood 1994: 86–7)

The post-industrial Left has as a major concern the effects of inequalities in the labour market on social cohesion and solidarity. As noted above, segregation and divisions in labour markets have significant implications for social inclusion and integration. André Gorz, in particular, has been vocal in support of the idea that individuals have a need to work in the public sphere as a mode of social insertion (Gorz 1989a). Following on from this it can be argued that individuals can have membership of and integration in a variety of communities without having full membership of society (Gorz 1992). Thus, for example, members of ethnic groups may well be members of a range of communities (geographical, religious, cultural, sexual orientation, etc.) without being fully integrated into society as a whole due to racial discrimination. Gorz proposes that work in the public sphere is the key form of social insertion as it gives individuals a specific form of identity and membership in relation to a broader social domain than the more restrictive concept of community. In this sense the inequalities highlighted by Modood provide a focal point for convergence and co-operation between anti-racists and the post-industrial Left. The latter, then, must call not only for the end of the 'work-based society' but must also argue for the fair redistribution of work between all individuals. This point recognises that the contemporary labour market in the new economy treats certain groups (notably ethnic minorities) in a less than equitable manner.[15] Not only is there inequality for migrant labour which is frequently used as an ample source of cheap labour without many of the rights of majority groups but resident ethnic minorities may also suffer from both higher levels of unemployment and state manipulation in 'lowering the reproductive costs of labour' (Pierson 1991: 89).

This section has placed considerable significance on feminist and anti-racist critiques of the welfare state for the development of post-industrial socialism. It is absolutely central to the latter that it embraces some of the less popular but wholly resonant perspectives on state welfare and attempts to influence a political agenda which is dominated by a somewhat limited triumvirate of ideological standpoints: namely, neo-liberal economic approaches; social democratic defences of humane, welfare capitalism; and neo-Marxist wholesale rejections of the welfare state. However, there is one further ideological perspective which has received little coverage in social policy literature and yet is highly pertinent to the post-industrial Left – political ecology.

Political ecology, welfare and post-industrialism

Political ecology is a highly complex political ideology which has not been addressed explicitly enough within social policy debates, although the main principles advocated by Greens have provided major questions for the future of welfare.[16] Green political thought has been largely ignored in the sphere of social policy, although more recently there has been a growing interest in this area (Skirbekk 1996; Kenny and Little 1995; Cahill 1995; George and Wilding 1994; Collinson 1996). This section will evaluate Green perspectives on welfare and attempt to differentiate between the ideas of political ecology and post-industrial socialism. This stands against the tendency among social policy analysts, and even some Green commentators, to conflate the two.[17]

Initially we can acknowledge that three features of the Green perspective have particular resonance for the post-industrial Left. First, it is important to note that the welfare of a society or an economy cannot be explained away by traditional economic indices such as GDP or GNP when those indices are focused on economic growth without taking into account the environmental damage (and consequently diswelfare) which economic growth engenders. Second, much of the strength of Green politics lies in the challenges to the traditional political order that it embodies and the notion that political change may well be reliant on popular movements as opposed to traditional political parties. In this sense key debates over social policies may well be taking place outside the domain of government and the state, despite being effectively marginalised from the mainstream forum. Finally, it is also pertinent to note that, against the proponents of the view that we have entered a 'post-industrial' era (Esping-Andersen 1993), the welfare state 'depends upon displacing the dysfunctions of economic growth upon the Third World, offering a national political solution which makes global problems of welfare still more severe' (Pierson 1991: 94).

Green political thought is characterised like other ideologies by the diversity of perspectives it embraces. Thus much analysis of it is primarily concerned with discerning different types of ecologism or environmentalism. Post-industrial socialism clearly draws much from within the Green tradition but it does so in an anthropocentric as opposed to ecocentric vein (Eckersley 1992). That is, rather than proceeding from the primacy of nature as a starting point, the essence of post-industrial socialism lies in Leftist humanism. Thus Pepper argues that 'we should proceed to ecology from social justice and not the other way round' (Pepper 1993: 3). This humanistic anthropocentrism is not compatible with the ideas of those who characterise ecologism as a coherent and strictly defined ideology in its own right (Dobson 1990). This is just one feature of the wide debate on Green thought about the internal coherence of ecologism, as the ecocentric/anthropocentric split is also mirrored by debates on deep versus shallow ecology, dark Green versus light Green theory and ultimately ecologism and environmentalism (Dobson 1990; Goodin 1992a; Kenny 1994).[18] Post-industrial socialism tends to fit into the weaker definition of each of these theoretical divides (shallow, light Green, environmentalist), although this does not necessarily indicate that it is any less radical than deep political ecology. What it does signify is that if we define political ecology in the narrow sense (Dobson 1990), then post-industrial socialism is clearly a different ideological perspective altogether. However, if a broader definition of ecologism is employed (Kenny 1994) then clearer points of convergence can be drawn. For our purposes Dobson's framework shall be used as an analytical tool, while still recognising Kenny's important point that drawing hard and fast lines on the ideological location of political ideas can be a dangerous game (Little 1996: 50–5; Kenny 1994: 223).

As mentioned above, it can be difficult clearly to discern what the Green theoretical perspective is on social policy (which is perhaps not surprising given that Greens tend to be primarily concerned with supposedly 'bigger' ideas and priorities), although Green parties have provided statements on social policy and the future of work in election manifestos (e.g. Green Party of Ireland 1989). Nevertheless, the absence of thorough debate on social policy in some of the major texts on Green theory suggests that this is an area where Greens have not been forthcoming enough. In one of the few contributions to ecologism and social policy, Ferris argues that

> there is as yet no consensually agreed green social policy although it is necessary to reconcile ecological and social concerns . . . Realistic green politics is premised on the belief that we do not have to sacrifice normative perspectives or basic ethical principles in order to explore possibilities of effective action in a threatened world. Greens need to think about means and ends and how they can be combined.
>
> (Ferris 1993: 157)

In other words, the Green critique of industrialism (in both capitalist and socialist forms) does not preclude the importance of debating Green alternatives to the institutions of industrial society and, of course, one of the most important of these is the welfare state. Indeed, as the progress of industrialism continues along with the ecological problems it engenders, it is increasingly incumbent on Greens to develop alternative social policies. Thus, as expressed by Ferris in an earlier contribution to this debate: 'Ecological concerns are now becoming social policy concerns. We do need urgently to develop these ideas in practical ways in social policy that will give rise to qualitative growth' (Ferris 1985: 71). Just as much mainstream social policy literature is littered with tokenistic references to 'the environment' or the 'Green movement' without full exposition of what the implications of environmental degradation entail, so political ecologists must be more explicit about the nitty-gritty of policy-making in a Green future.

This signals an area where divergence between post-industrial socialism and ecologism is clear. The former has been active in providing potential alternatives to the present social policy whereas Greens have been more reticent. Wall, for example, says much about the future of Green economics without elaborating greatly on the relationship between economic and social policy. Similarly, Tindale, from a much less radical approach, discusses the economy purely in terms of taxation without relating economic issues to the future of welfare (Tindale 1994). In attempting to demonstrate that the environment is a natural issue of concern for social democrats, he fails to deal with the issue of social policy, telling us instead that there is a dilemma on the Left over 'whether redistribution is possible in the absence of rapid economic growth' (Tindale 1994: 204). In short, he signals a central problem in the thinking of the Left and Greens without fully discussing the options for social policy.[19] At least Wall does provide an illustration of a key feature of the future Green economy (which, however, is rather different from Gorz's view on the economy) and, in comparison to Tindale, he is aware of the major upheavals that ecologism entails if carried through to the full extent. Wall (1990: 80) states that 'Ecology is incompatible with the market' and continues by explaining 'how to smash capitalism gently'. In Chapter 1 we saw how Gorz envisages a continued (though strictly limited) role for markets in a post-industrial socialist society, which indicates a rather different perspective from Wall's. Indeed, the latter has only one very short paragraph on basic income schemes (which are examined in Chapters 5 and 6) as a possible Green alternative for welfare, despite the fact that his book is entitled *Getting There: Steps to a Green Society*. If the road to a Green society does not develop a coherent and thoroughgoing set of social policies, then it does not appear to be leading us very far.

A notable exception to the rule in Green political theory in analysing social policy is Alain Lipietz (1993). He is most commonly known as a Green analyst of the 'post-Fordist' economy but he goes beyond this to point out the implications of the new economy and ecological concerns for state welfare. Although his ideas on the future of welfare are not completely resonant with post-industrial socialist approaches (as we shall see in later chapters), his Green critique of the welfare state offers much in the process of defining the key foundations of post-industrial socialist social policy. Like Gorz, Lipietz sees the welfare state as an institution which is intrinsically linked to notions of full employment (in terms of the family wage, at least) and economic growth fostered by Fordism. With the demise of the latter and the consequent unlikelihood of the former, a new vision of a 'welfare community' is required which encompasses less human time being spent in the sphere of work (Lipietz 1993: 80). This supposes a new 'ecological compromise' to replace Fordist organicism:

> Fordism had at its disposal a powerful tool of solidarity – the welfare state, social security, various welfare benefits and allowances. These have been attacked, rightly, as bureaucratic. The alternative compromise must take on 'individual' aspirations to be responsible for one's affairs, to see things through to their conclusion. To establish an 'individual organicist' paradigm is the challenge facing us.
>
> (Lipietz 1993: 92)

Thus the essential key to understanding Lipietz's perspective on the welfare state is that it is viewed as a compromise which he believes is the basis of any welfare system. The capitalist welfare state, however, was a compromise between capital and labour that was reliant on a significant majority of people working, which was deemed the 'normal' means of accessing a reasonable standard of living. In this sense those who were reliant on welfare benefits were deemed to be living in an 'abnormal' way. For Lipietz, this is the opposite of a welfare community, rather it is anti-communitarian, especially as access to employment became less open with the demise of Fordism which led to much more disaffection in general with those who had to claim benefits. In short, the welfare state was founded on Fordist principles which were no longer applicable after the mid-1970s. In the Fordist era, of course, work was more abundant (though mainly for men) and this disguised the 'bizarre rule' that people should be working or available for work before recourse to benefits. Lipietz believes that the end of full employment (as it was understood in the post-war era) points to the growing inability of the welfare state to perform the task allotted to it. This outlook is similar to that held by members of the post-industrial Left such as Gorz, which should not be surprising given that Lipietz is fairly moderate when it comes to the full spectrum of Green political thought. In analysing Lipietz's critique of the Fordist welfare state, there appear to be certain areas of convergence with earlier neo-Marxist crisis theories, although the former is clearly more aware of the environmental impact of the Keynesian welfare state (Gough 1995: 215). Lipietz provides fruitful ground for post-industrial socialism in demonstrating that a future welfare settlement cannot be uncritically based upon full employment as it is traditionally understood, which is at best an anachronism in the current era and at worst a pipedream or homage to productivist economic growth that can lead to 'social exclusions and the accumulation of ecological tensions and international imbalances' (Lipietz 1994: 345).

Conclusion

This section has focused on a variety of critiques of the welfare state which all, to a greater or lesser extent, have some bearing on the post-industrial Left, not only in analysing the welfare state, but also in developing a radical alternative to present arrangements. Thus the coverage here has not been intended as a thorough critique of each ideological viewpoint or an expression of ideological coherence within the different critiques involved. Rather, the exercise involved in this chapter has been the identification of certain ideas and perspectives on the welfare state which can be used in new ways by post-industrial socialists. In this sense we can see the theoretical origins of ideas which can be fused into a new, coherent critique of the welfare state which can then be applied to fresh ideas on the future of social policy. The point we have reached so far, then, can be summarised as follows:

- Post-industrial socialism is a doctrine which sees the future of Leftist politics in opposing the methods of industrial capitalism and the economic and social principles embodied by the latter.
- In terms of the welfare state, this means rejecting notions of traditionally understood full employment, unregulated economic growth, bureaucratic and intrusive welfarism, and the strong links between work and the payment of benefits.
- The neo-liberal tradition has contributed to this insofar as it has signalled the importance of economic policy and the ineffectiveness of the welfare state in reaching the desired objectives. However, the overall thrust of neo-liberalism is rejected because of the neglect of social policy and the glorification of the market with scant regard for market outcomes and their negative effect on social cohesion and solidarity.
- Neo-Marxism is instructive in terms of highlighting the ongoing contradictions and crises of welfare capitalism, although it should be clearer in signalling that a future socialism might also experience crises. Like neo-liberals, neo-Marxists have outlined the failure of the welfare state in achieving radical socialist objectives and the inability of social democratic governments to provide a humane face of capitalism. This entails a new direction for socialist politics beyond the welfare state.
- Feminist and anti-racist analyses suggest that the welfare state is

58

extremely partial and that critics of the Left and Right have not been perceptive enough in understanding the effects of the welfare state on women and ethnic minority groups. They provide a stark reminder for the post-industrial Left that debates on the future of social policy cannot only be located in terms of class but need to understand other social fragmentations along the lines of ethnicity, gender, disability, and so on. These perspectives also bring into focus prominent issues such as the nature of work and their impact on social policy debates.

- Greens, though generally reticent about social welfare, have much to say on how we define welfare itself. They point to several features of the welfare state, such as economic growth and industrial methods, which are harmful to the environment and, therefore, harmful for all (including humans) who live in a specific environment. While Greens need to be more explicit about the future of social policy, they do recognise that debates about welfare are international and that individual nations cannot solve the diswelfare caused by international capital.

From the above it should be clear that the roots of post-industrial socialism are manifold and that the fusion of the ideas outlined above gives a fairly unique character to the post-industrial Left. Again this is not to say that it is necessarily an ideology in itself, far from it, but that it is a clear variant within the broad church of socialism. It has a distinctive critique of the welfare state and welfare capitalism in general which borrows much from a variety of ideological backgrounds without losing sight of primary objectives such as solidarity, equality, mutualism and individual liberty. From this foundational point we can begin to build a picture of what the post-industrial Left has in mind for the future of social welfare. Before analysing different policy proposals towards the end of this book, it is important to look at two key principles which form the basis of those proposals: namely, the creation of a coherent theory of socialist citizenship and a conceptualisation of basic human needs. For the post-industrial Left, without an understanding of these two concepts, we can have little understanding of where we are trying to get to. In short, we need an idea of what principles post-industrial socialism embraces if we are to begin to imagine a future for welfare that understands new social and economic realities.

3

TOWARDS SOCIALIST
CITIZENSHIP

The debate over citizenship, which was one of the foundational points of reference for the formation of the welfare state, has recently re-emerged in reaction to the changing social policies of governments throughout the world and the growing resonance of socialist, feminist and anti-racist critiques of the rights and obligations that citizenship was thought to embody.[1] The crises of the Fordist–Keynesian welfare state and the failure of government policies to deal with those crises have led to a re-evaluation of the meaning of citizenship, particularly with regard to social rights. For the post-industrial Left, the new citizenship debate provides an opportunity to move beyond traditional views of political, civil and social rights and attempt to introduce new economic rights which might breed greater independence. Moreover, the debate also generates the possibility of clarifying what obligations should be reciprocally attached to the rights of citizenship and how concrete these obligations should be. Thus the resurgence of discourses on citizenship enables post-industrial socialists to outline the implications that the end of 'work-based society' could have for the future shape of state welfare and, consequently, the potential developments on the horizon for a new socialist citizenship.

Rights and citizenship

The most conventional method of approaching the citizenship debate is to analyse the work of T. H. Marshall, who had a profound influence on British sociology and social policy in the immediate post-war years.[2] For Marshall, the basis of citizenship was to be found in a triumvirate of rights: civil, political and social. Civil rights referred to the legal safeguards that protected individual liberties with regard to speech, movement and religion, the right to own property and, most importantly, the protection of these rights by law. These features had mainly evolved in the eighteenth century and were highly significant because they implemented 'the right to defend and assert all one's rights on terms of equality with others and by due process of law' (Marshall 1994: 173). Political rights, which he deemed to have their root in the nineteenth century, involved the extension of the franchise to allow individuals to exercise influence over local and national government through their vote and the right to stand for political office. The social element of citizenship rights, which Marshall associated with the twentieth century, involved the development of social welfare measures such as social, health and educational services which would allow individuals to 'live the life of a civilized being according to the standards prevailing in the society' (Marshall 1994: 173).[3] Importantly, the equal extension of these rights of citizenship would result in class-abatement whereby inequalities of resources between classes would not result in conflict because equal citizenship would generate equal status despite inequalities of outcome. Thus, as Pinker has observed, 'Marshall's model of society does not . . . preclude the occurrence of conflict or of unsystematic aspects of social life' (Pinker 1995: 104). Indeed, as several commentators have argued, the conflicts associated with the inequalities of capitalism were unlikely to be solved easily as only the social rights of welfare actually required any sort of compromise between labour and capital. Civil and political rights were actually conducive to the systemic reproduction of capitalism (Turner 1993a).

Marshall's work is clearly relevant to any analysis of developments in social policy but its importance in terms of socialism is not so clear. Indeed, although his work is often identified with the social democratic welfare state, he appears to owe much to the 'new liberal' tradition (Pierson 1991; Pinker 1995). Marshall believed that citizenship could be achieved in a market-based society despite the inevitable inequalities inherent in capitalism. This would be achieved by the state intervening to offset the worst of these inequalities, which leads us to a classic defence of a pluralistic mixed economy. This had not been fully achieved in Marshall's time due to the failure of the state in reining in the interests of capital but he believed that the welfare state and the new social rights it engendered would lead to genuine citizenship (Heater 1990: 101; Pinker 1995: 113). Clearly, and not surprisingly given the period in which his most influential work was written, Marshall's ideas are linked closely with the workerist welfare state which emerged in the post-war era. The demise of the welfare state as a key reproductive aid to advanced capitalism leads to questions regarding the applicability of his theoretical ideas to the future of social policy if we are entering a post-industrial era. However, that should not diminish the idea that civil, political and social rights are key features of how future citizenship should be encapsulated.

Pierson notes how Marshall offers few pointers as to how to generate a new universal citizenship which would imply 'a state which is both strengthened and more circumscribed – a constitutionally self-limiting state. In this context, the real difficulty is to establish how citizens are to exercise effective control over a state from which their capacities as citizens derive' (Pierson 1991: 204).

The task ahead is to look at Marshall's conception of these rights and to evaluate their resonance in his own era and then assess their usefulness for the post-industrial Left. From this we can begin to outline a new post-industrial socialist theory of citizenship which goes beyond the more limited ideas of Marshall, with particular regard to economic rights, and explore the liberatory potential of the concept of citizenship.[4] This entails the idea of broadening citizenship to encapsulate a socialist political project because, as Clarke (1994: 28) notes, 'Marshall regarded citizenship as a dynamic concept but did not see its full potential for human emancipation'.

Critics of Marshall have often pointed to his optimistic belief in class-abatement and the abstract notions which underpin his concept of citizenship. Twine, for example, notes how Marshall confuses opportunities and rights, a confusion which obscures how formal rights can be anything but substantive. Thus 'in the same way that there is no right to property, so there is no right to employment. There are, however, opportunities to own property or to be employed' (Twine 1994: 36). Twine correctly points to the centrality of paid work in industrial societies if individuals are to gain independence and the economic welfare which is central to social inclusion. In other words, if individuals are to be citizens (full members of society), they require a certain level of economic well-being to be able to participate fully in social and political life. In this sense Marshall's conception of citizenship rights is too abstract to be useful to concrete analyses of what citizenship could entail in the future. Certainly, civil, political and social rights are vital features of citizenship but a fourth dimension which recognises economic welfare should also be introduced to the equation, particularly as opportunities in the labour markets of the new economy have profound effects on all of Marshall's rights of citizenship. This signals the complex relationship between citizenship and economic conditions. The former, while not determined by the latter, is reliant on appropriate distribution of economic resources to ensure the type of egalitarian relations on which the notion of citizenship is fundamentally based. For Marshall, the right to work was a civil right (Marshall 1994: 174) which would ensure some distribution of economic resources. But, clearly, even in the immediate post-war years, there has been no civil right to work since the eighteenth century, let alone more recently when unemployment has become a permanent feature of advanced capitalist economies. It is for this reason that post-industrial socialists view economic rights as a separate category from Marshall's other rights. A similar perspective is adopted by Twine, who observes that 'it is not appropriate to include a labour contract as a civil right. The right to a labour contract is in reality not a right but an opportunity' (Twine 1994: 108). In this sense, the development of social citizenship that supposedly accompanied the rise of the welfare state should not be seen as the final stage of development in citizenship and we have not witnessed 'the end of the history of citizenship' (Van Steenbergen 1994: 3). Where Marshall saw citizenship as 'a non-economic concept' (Dahrendorf 1994: 13), the post-industrial Left believe citizenship to be peripheral in generating an egalitarian project if it ignores economic circumstances.

A different critique of Marshallian citizenship rights is formulated by Habermas, who questions the nature of rights (both positive and negative) in liberal democracies. His perspective is based upon the limitations of rights discourses against the powers of the state. Thus conferring individuals with a variety of rights does not necessarily entail giving them the power of autonomous choice over how those rights are experienced or acted upon. Abstract rights can be granted and legally located in social institutions without developing individual autonomy or making states particularly democratic. In the words of Habermas:

> Liberal or negative and social or positive rights can . . . be conferred by a paternalistic authority. In principle, then, the rule of law and the welfare state can exist without the concomitant existence of democracy. Liberal and social rights remain ambiguous in Western countries where all three categories of rights are institutionalized . . . [R]ights of individual freedom and social security can just as well facilitate a privatist retreat from citizenship and a particular 'clientelization' of the citizen's role.
>
> (Habermas 1994: 31)

Habermas is articulating one of the key concerns with citizenship which is articulated in terms of formal rights. In practice formal rights may shift the burden of responsibility for decision-making from publicly accountable bodies and institutions to individuals with little access to the decision-making process. According to the formal rights discourse, individuals are conferred individual decision-making power despite the fact that individuals may not have sufficient resources to exercise their formal powers. This raises a dilemma for a post-industrial Left which is seeking to regenerate notions of citizenship. It can either abandon notions of rights which would make expressions of citizenship extremely difficult or it can attempt to outline policies designed to make rights and obligations more substantive and tangible. The latter perspective has been adhered to more often, given that a substantive notion of citizenship can help to outline strategies for social integration and inclusion, and may explore methods of empowering communities and individuals against the centralisation of power in national or international systems. This begins the process of developing a democratic civil society which can exercise decision-making powers. This would need to subvert the condition engendered by contemporary citizenship whereby rights, rather than helping individuals to interact in the public sphere, actually dislocate them in the private sphere with little power to influence decision-making. According to Habermas, this process of clientelisation becomes all the more prevalent as

> the economy and the state apparatus – which have been institutionalized in terms of the same rights [as citizens] – develop a systemic autonomy and push citizens into the periphery of organizational membership. As self-regulating systems, economy and administration tend to cut themselves off from their environments and obey only their internal imperatives of money and power. They no longer fit into the model of a self-determining community of citizens.
>
> (Habermas 1994: 31–2)

This builds upon the earlier Habermasian notion of the 'colonisation of the lifeworld', whereby the rationality of social systems such as the economy and administration expand their own productivist rationalities into all spheres of everyday life unencumbered by popular democratic control. This leads Lodziak to comment that unless 'we seize the chance to develop social networks and communities that facilitate self-determination (autonomy) and collective self-determination (democracy) we will be subjected to further encroachments from the social system' (Lodziak 1995: 22). This statement neatly encapsulates the general standpoint of post-industrial socialists who want to limit spheres imbued with systemic economic rationality and open up new realms where individuals and communities can exercise greater control over democratically invigorated areas of civil society. This involves reconsidering our conception of rights and, from a Leftist perspective, solidifying the formality of liberal rights into materially substantive socialist rights of citizenship which encompass access to the public sphere rather than the privatistic effects of liberal notions of citizenship rights (Gorz 1989a: 140; Lodziak 1995:

73-91). In this sense the debate is moving beyond the limited parameters associated with more traditional approaches, such as that of Marshall.

Rethinking rights

Post-industrial socialists are keen to delineate rights and obligations for individuals, communities and states more concretely than has previously been the case in liberal democratic societies. It is only through this kind of systematic thinking about what rights and obligations will actually mean in practice that we will be able to defend individual and collective autonomy from the excesses of state power and the economic rationality of markets. In this sense civil rights must be defined in such a way that the legal constraints on individuals *and the state* are clearly evident. Political rights and the right to participation also need to be identified if we are to be able to locate decision-making power and accountability. In liberal democratic notions of citizenship these two types of rights have been enshrined in such a way that they reinforce rather than question the systemic nature of capitalism. For example, civil rights have been used to frame the right (or, more properly, the opportunity) to own property which is functional for capitalist reproduction. Moreover, they are primarily concerned with 'the capacity to enter market exchanges as independent and self-sufficient agents . . . If such rights are the core of citizenship, then citizenship will consolidate class inequalities' (Barbalet 1993: 37). Elsewhere, Barbalet has observed that: 'Civil rights in citizenship consolidate capitalist relationships . . . and therefore capitalist class power' (Barbalet 1988: 33). Similarly, political rights to vote or stand for election help to reinforce the representative nature of liberal democracies. In most liberal democracies there may well be a large degree of equality in terms of the value of each individual vote, but this should not lead to a glossing over of the effects of political rights in reproducing representative democracy. By highlighting the inadequacies of conventional rights discourses, we can then outline new perspectives on social and economic rights which can engender a more concrete and equal understanding of citizenship.

Autonomy and civil rights

Civil rights are important for the post-industrial Left because they can be used to defend individual autonomy and outline individual and state obligations which can be legally enshrined. In this sense civil rights need not be defined as negative rights of liberty as they are in liberal democracies and in Marshall's work (Habermas 1994: 30). If civil rights promote the principle of individual autonomy – that is, the right to self-determine one's activities – then they become much more positive phenomena. As noted earlier, in liberal democracies civil rights such as the right to property are really framed as protective laws that endow opportunities to do certain things without actually embodying an attempt at achieving equal status as Marshall intended.[5] One can be equally treated in the eyes of the law without having equal access to the ownership of property which, in advanced capitalist societies, may well be seen as having a bearing on social status. Currently, as Hindess observes, the 'extension of civil rights to most of the adult population does little to overcome the effects of major economic inequalities' (Hindess 1993: 25). Post-industrial socialism comprises an attempt at providing a broad framework for positive freedoms which could be enshrined in civil rights. With the idea of positive freedoms, then, equal status appears on the horizon, though not nearly close enough because rights to do something do not necessarily entail self-determination. In other words, the legal autonomy of an individual to do something may be curtailed by socio-economic circumstances such as the lack of resources (both financial and temporal) and the absence of certain social services (e.g. state nursery provision).

The post-industrial Left, while recognising the constraints imposed by traditional civil rights discourses, believes that legal protections are important in the sense, for example, that individuals should be defended from violence against them by the state or other individuals. However, we must also note that traditional rights discourses can be seen to be exclusionary because, in defining who has civil rights, we are also defining who does not have them. This scenario is unacceptable as it immediately throws up a barrier to social integration and may be used as a means of discriminating against people on grounds of culture, nationality, religion, and so on. Post-industrial socialists, in declaring the universality of rights, need not be prescriptive about how those rights are exercised. There is no reason why declarations of universal rights should mitigate against people who have different national identities, especially in an era when transnational mobility is becoming more prevalent. Kallscheuer argues that the 'libertarian Left' should engage with Europe as an 'open social space', abandon differences between citizens and aliens and seek 'a civil (not national) definition of European citizenship' (Kallscheuer 1994: 136). This necessitates a very different conception of the politics of rights in which the latter are envisaged as universal in a new political culture which promotes inclusion and integration. While such a transformation of political culture is a difficult task to envisage, some commentators point out that large swaths of people 'have become alienated from organised politics' (Lodziak 1995: 13) and, although it will be a difficult process, that there is potential for a new oppositional culture based on the expansion of a culture of autonomy (Lodziak 1995: 92–113). Lodziak contends that anti-systemic social movements have a central role to play in developing a culture for autonomy:

> [A] culture for autonomy is the foundation for a culture of opposition. A culture for autonomy becomes a culture of opposition as the continuing expansion of the sphere of autonomy increasingly necessitates contestation against the capitalist system. Bonds of solidarity, which develop as a consequence of people's practical involvement with each other on autonomous projects, are vital in sustaining participation in contestatory politics.
>
> (Lodziak 1995: 118)

Political rights and participation in the public sphere

The necessity of developing a new political culture is an arduous process but it is not one that should be disregarded out of hand. Ideas which question productivist assumptions, the current politics of time, the changing nature of work and welfare, and the malaise within the organised political system are dealing with profoundly important political issues. Moreover, these issues are grounded in the lived experience of individuals, far as that might be from the mainstream culture of organised politics. While the existence and primacy of these issues does not suggest that significant change is imminent, it does provide potential on which radical policy proposals can be built. Importantly, it designates sound grounds on which to premise a change in political participation and the regeneration of democracy. It links in with some radical communitarian proposals for democratising civil society and it has profound implications for what the post-industrial Left is to propose for the future of political rights.

Political rights as understood in the traditional liberal theories of rights are extremely limited from the post-industrial socialist perspective, based as they are in the reproduction of dominant models of representative democracy. The notions of voting rights and the opportunity to stand in electoral contests are far too limited to provide a political backdrop to a democratic system which is directed towards individual autonomy, self-determining communities and rejuvenated civil society. Liberal political rights, on the other hand, are based upon very limited ideas of political activity, the abdication of responsibility to various strata of government and centralised decision-making procedures. They form an ingredient in the recipe of increasing privatism which is 'a form of social and political withdrawal. People get on with their private lives while the powers that be get on with the important matters. The reproduction of the capitalist system is secured in privatism' (Lodziak 1995: 68). Privatism is not to be seen as the fault of individuals behaving in a privatistic manner, as most people do at times in advanced capitalist societies, but rather as a systemic requirement of advanced capitalism which manages to generate social and political alienation among the vast majority of the population. The bottom line is that, if individuals are deprived of influence over the decision-making process, then disillusionment with the whole domain of organised politics develops. This suits the needs of the participants in organised politics which can then be conducted in a rarefied atmosphere that does not correspond with the lived reality of most people. Thus, for example, trade unions, which performed a central role in the representation of labour in industrial society, have become increasingly detached from the experience of those who have been worst affected by the requirements of the new economy.

The concept of political rights opposed here is one where accountable decision-making is actually undermined by the rights that are granted, that is, where representative democracy becomes an end in itself at the expense of allowing individuals and communities to take some of the decisions that affect them directly. The post-industrial Left approaches rights as a concept as much related to equality as to liberty. Thus it is not enough to have the opportunity to vote or stand for election if we do not have the equal chance to take autonomous control of our own lives or to influence decision-making in our communities. The liberal assumption that there is an equal political community needs to be questioned. Moreover, when it comes to welfare, it is vital that individuals and communities have the ability to influence social policies which affect them. The right to vote does not necessarily confer that ability in the sense that 'politics has gradually become a matter of administration', which in turn undermines 'the status of [the] citizen and [denies] the republican meat of such a status' (Habermas 1994: 30). The long and short of this scenario is that organised politics has become a void when it comes to meaningful political debate. Thus, while Deakin is close to the mark when stating that 'democracy . . . has a potentially crucial relationship to welfare', he is overly optimistic in stating that the vote is 'potentially important in helping to decide the direction of welfare policies by giving the citizens the opportunity to articulate their demands' (Deakin 1994: 14). This is a very limited understanding of political rights which suggests that genuine power can be exercised by the vote. Certainly, minimal accountability can be experienced through the vote, but it is a far cry from the notion of individual autonomy in the sense of self-determination or collective self-determination for communities. The analysis of citizenship too often focuses on social policy in isolation from civil and political rights which can lead to statements such as 'the existence of political rights *per se* is not in dispute' (Deakin 1994: 213). While there is a virtually universal franchise in such countries as the United Kingdom, this does not necessarily entail a thorough conception of political rights or democracy as a whole (Arblaster 1994). In other words, 'a recognition that universal suffrage and representative institutions can enhance the opportunities and conditions of the working class need not deny that these same institutions can stabilize the existing social order and serve its dominant class by helping to channel and reduce popular pressure and conflict' (Barbalet 1988: 83).

The post-industrial Left, then, adopts a perspective whereby there is a clear connection in the overall scheme of things between different types of rights which *together* help to develop socialist citizenship. Meehan describes this type of analysis as 'Aristotelian and/or idealist' and suggests that it entails the view that 'individuals are human beings only when they belong to a community and, being essentially political, their humanity is expressed when they take part in constructing and maintaining their community' (Meehan 1993: 6). Certainly, post-industrial socialists can be regarded as 'radical communitarians' (Hughes and Little 1996), insofar as theorists such as Offe and Gorz are concerned with the development of collective self-determination in sub-state units such as communities. They adhere to Meehan's description of this 'idealist' theoretical standpoint:

> The good society is not only the same as participatory society but it is also a moral order of well-being and conviviality. Private interests . . . and public interests cannot exist distinctly from one another since they converge on the common human need for the good society in all its dimensions. Political rights to discharge public duties entail trying to find a fair distribution of social justice. . . . social rights are not an instrument for the pursuit of personal ends but are both the cause and reflection of a solidaristic moral order.
>
> (Meehan 1993: 6)

In this sense the minimalist nature of liberal political rights is inadequate for the kind of broad conception (often expressed in 'grand narratives') of the interdependence of rights in post-industrial socialist thought. Just as liberal civil rights are primarily concerned with negative freedoms based on legal protection rather than a theoretical principle such as autonomy, so liberal political rights are concerned with the formal ability to express political beliefs rather than concrete principles of autonomous political actions. As noted earlier, in effect, liberal civil and political rights do nothing to undermine traditional hierarchical political culture and have little impact on the generation of an emancipatory oppositional culture. The next step in our evaluation of post-industrial socialist approaches to citizenship is to examine the nature of social rights and to assess whether they hold potential for the development of oppositional culture.

From social rights to economic rights

Social rights are commonly treated as the most controversial dimension of Marshall's triumvirate of rights because, unlike negative civil and political rights, there is a positive dimension to the notion of social rights. Rather than enshrining opportunities to engage in certain activities, social rights imply an obligation on the part of the state to ensure the well-being of members of society. This asks fundamental questions of the capitalist system in a way that is not comprised in liberal civil and political rights. In Twine's words, 'social rights are a direct challenge to a social class stratified society wherein most people must sell their labour power in the labour market in order to obtain a standard of living' (Twine 1994: 102). Despite this, it can be dangerous to compartmentalise social rights as completely different entities from civil and political rights because this opens up space for neo-liberal arguments which believe the latter need not interfere with markets whereas the former certainly would and, therefore, should be opposed. On the other hand, if we develop a theory of social rights informed indirectly by a thorough theory of human needs (as is attempted in the next chapter), then social rights might acquire similar status as traditional liberal rights. Thus, as Plant observes, 'the provision of resources to meet basic needs has to be seen as a duty on government in the same way as the protection of civil rights is a duty' (Plant 1985: 28). Indeed, if post-industrial socialists advocate autonomy as the guiding theoretical principle of civil rights, then it is incumbent on those defining the content of social rights to embed autonomy in social policy debates. Similarly, as Twine argues, there is an interdependence between social rights and political rights as the latter open up spaces about debate over the former. If post-industrial socialists enshrine autonomy (experienced as self-determination) as their basis for rights discourses, then political rights must permit individuals to take more control and responsibility for their own lives, as must social rights.

Just as the liberal rights in Marshall's triumvirate have been criticised by the post-industrial Left for their rather limited nature, so social rights are challenged for providing limited social welfare benefits rather than concrete economic measures which can enable all individuals to partake fully in social life. If social rights are designed to reflect our social inter-dependence as individuals (Twine 1994; Ferris 1985), then the limited availability of state welfare benefits hardly encapsulates social rights as too many benefits are means tested and discretionary, which must disqualify them from being characterised as rights. Thus Ferris claims that:

> The social rights that Marshall identified turned out to be not so much the 'universal rights to real income' but provisional and highly circumscribed obligations accepted by the political man-agers as necessary to secure consent and to meet certain forms of manifest need created by high intensity market society. The circumscribed and provisional nature of these 'rights' is very clear when we consider the wilful legal and administrative com-plexity of social security provisions.
>
> (Ferris 1985: 53)

Thus Ferris views social rights in the Marshallian sense as a misnomer which does not really encompass universalistic principles. In comparison with political rights, for example, this claim can be verified by looking at the limited number of adult people excluded from voting and the num-bers, including some of the very worst off, who are excluded from receiv-ing various welfare benefits. Thus claiming benefits can be an arduous and stigmatising process in which people have to go to extreme lengths to explain their eligibility, only to suffer much criticism for 'scrounging from the state' and not getting a job. This kind of procedure cannot be equated with universal social rights let alone an embodiment of social jus-tice underpinned by rights. For this reason Barbalet states that Marshall's equation of social rights and social policy is 'historically limited . . . and logically flawed' (Barbalet 1988: 64). In this sense social rights discourses have all too often been subsumed by broader debates about welfare pro-vision, and the nature of rights themselves has become obscured.[6] For post-industrial socialists, social rights should be clearly outlined so that the state has responsibility for universal payments to each individual who contributes to the generation of social wealth, that is, every individ-ual who works for wages in the public sphere. Moreover, every individual should be provided with the opportunity to make their contribution to the social whole by enshrining an economic right to work for wages. However, this undertaking can only be facilitated by reducing working hours for everyone in order to allow work to be distributed more equitably. Even the reduction of working hours for everyone would not provide sufficient work for all in an era when the number of meaningful jobs is contracting (Offe 1985). For this reason, theorists such as Gorz suggest that in this case there should be a social right to an income for periods when one is not working. In this sense, then, where social rights were originally developed along with the growth of the industrial system, so the potential advent of post-industrial society allows (and indeed necessitates) a thorough rethinking of social rights. Furthermore, when the primary means of achieving economic well-being in industrial society, work for wages, becomes less widespread, then a case arises for developing a social right to economic well-being which takes into account the unavailability of sufficient jobs to allow all individuals to take care of their own welfare themselves. For the post-industrial Left, then, the social side of citizenship should encompass an economic right to work for wages and a social right for individuals to universal state welfare benefits regardless of whether they are working for wages at any given time. This is a fundamental reversal of welfare provisions in work-based societies because

> the social democratic project of defending (on the European continent) a contributory and incomes-graduated system of transfers is based upon not citizens', but employees' rights and duties. Mandatory contributions to the systems of old age pensions, health insurance and unemployment insurance are (within upper and lower limits) tied to the legal status of being an employee, and benefits are allocated (with the limited exception of the case of health services) in accordance with the duration of employment and the income earned during that employment.
>
> (Offe 1992: 70)

Obviously, then, the post-industrial socialist perspective on citizenship entails an absolute rejection of social rights based solely upon work for wages. In other words, the development of social 'rights' in the welfare state cannot be the basis of social justice in an era when meaningful work for wages is becoming increasingly scarce (Offe 1985: 144–5). The post-industrial Left advocates individual economic rights which exceed previous conceptions of industrial democracy that concerned rights to organise collectively to influence relations in the workplace (Turner 1993a: 7; Held 1989: 201). Economic rights are different from conceptions of industrial rights (Barbalet 1988; Meehan 1993) precisely because they are based upon universal economic well-being regardless of work performed. In this way economic rights, coupled with universal social rights, can be viewed as a foundational post-industrial socialist move beyond industrial rights. Where industrial rights can be defined as 'the rights of individuals permitting (and perhaps enabling) their collective action and organization' through the 'institutional bases of . . . trade unions and similar associations of employees' (Barbalet 1988: 26), the post-industrial Left sees social and economic rights as a more developed version of individual rights which encompasses the right to work and the right to periods away from work without losing an income from the state. Whereas Barbalet sees industrial rights as non-individualistic and non-obligatory, André Gorz points out that citizenship rights and duties are inextricably linked and that if we propose that individuals should have a right to work for wages then we must counter that with an obligation to work in the public sphere. Thus the concept of rights entails not only the protection of individuals but also the duties of individuals to others. Gorz argues that there

> can be no rights without corresponding obligations. My duty is the basis of my rights and to relieve me of all duties is to deny me the status of a person having rights. Rights and duties are always two sides of the same coin: my rights are the duties of others towards me; they imply my duties towards these others.
>
> (Gorz 1989a: 207)

This does not mean that we should have an obligation to work full-time throughout our lives – this would be impossible anyway as there would be insufficient work to go around – but rather that we can work towards the creation of social wealth intermittently, while also working voluntarily in communities and engaging in autonomous activities. Thus Lodziak argues that our 'obligation to work . . . can be fulfilled at times and periods in our lives when it most suits. Working time does not have to be continuous – it can be intermittent in any number of ways' (Lodziak 1995: 103). Clearly, then, the key feature of the post-industrial socialist conception of economic rights is not just the right to work in the public sphere towards the creation of social wealth but, and just as importantly, the right not to work, that is, the right for individuals to spend time pursuing non-wage-based activities. Thus, rather than viewing economic rights as the state providing opportunities for people to work, the post-industrial Left advocates substantive economic rights which could help to change the way we understand all our activities. A reduction in working hours would provide a scenario whereby civil rights based upon autonomy could be actualised and open up spaces for individuals to participate in their communities and act upon their political right to partake in the decision-making process.

Obligations of citizenship

The notion of obligation in the citizenship equation is both complex and relatively neglected when compared to discussion of rights (Saunders 1993: 77).[7] It is a slippery concept around which the Left treads carefully as it can potentially be manipulated by the Right to introduce conditionality into the welfare equation and thereby to undermine universalist features of citizenship (Roche 1992). However, there is considerable value in approaching citizenship from the perspective of duties because it enables us to outline what needs to be done to achieve socialist aims. Thus Bellamy suggests that a 'framework of duties . . . provides the basis for a participatory form of citizenship in which we collectively decide on our legal rights through the exercise of our civic obligations' (Bellamy 1993a: 69). This approach is particularly useful when attempting to theorise policy proposals for future society in which obligations are to be much more substantive than 'to contribute taxation to a state system of provision' (Turner 1993b: xi). The post-industrial Left tends to use the concept of obligation or duties in a fairly abstract way to enshrine the principle of interdependence in social relations. In this sense the duties attached to rights may become 'indeterminate' without losing sight of the fact that 'rights cannot be maintained without a network of duties attached to them, some of which may be practically closer and more central to, others more distant from, the nature of each right' (Freeden 1991: 78–9). Freeden points to the lack of symmetry between rights and duties and the implicit dangers of 'schematic oversimplification' in discourses on rights and obligations such as is the case with neo-conservative 'workfare' policies (Mead 1985; Pascall 1993). However, he does suggest a solution whereby communities can act as mediators in determining and concretising the rights and duties of individuals which certainly suggests an element of collective self-determination. Thus he suggests that:

> The system of mutual dependence gives rise to expectations and kinds of conduct without which human action and survival are inconceivable and that system may conveniently be described and shored up (though not solely) in terms of rights and duties. The very idea of rights and duties . . . reflects the existence of associations between and among people. As social

creatures human beings may claim rights not only against each other but against society in general, just as society will recipro-cate by claiming rights against individuals.

(Freeden 1991: 80)

It is clear from this analysis that a claim of rights implies a reciprocal, though not necessarily direct, obligation on the part of others to respect those rights. As an abstract liberal principle this has relevance for the post-industrial Left but the nature of duties expounded by Freeden remains open to practical interpretation. This is the point at which the Left has to tackle the difficult task of creating a redefinition of obligation and responsibility as part of a strategy of rethinking the notion of social-ist citizenship. Thus Harris argues that 'rather than being squeamish, the left should . . . try to design mechanisms to "encourage" obligations fairly for all (not just welfare recipients)' (Harris 1996: 1894). Post-industrial socialism is concerned primarily with individual and collective self-determination, but theorists such as Gorz are aware that the condi-tions under which autonomy may flourish must be underpinned by a clear understanding of the reciprocal duties between society, community and the individual. At present most Western European welfare regimes link welfare provision with the duty to seek employment which in itself is inherently exclusionary and assumes that paid work should be the pri-mary human activity. Gorz, on the other hand, believes in an obligation for *all* citizens to contribute to the generation of social wealth which can then be redistributed according to the principles of social justice which the post-industrial Left employs. At the same time, each individual has a duty to perform work for wages for a *limited* amount of time to enable enough work in the public sphere to be available for everyone. Thus he believes that the obligation to perform socially useful work is the key means of generating *social* inclusion in the sense that inclusion and mem-bership are only really facilitated by participation in any sphere of life (Gorz 1992). Other forms of work, such as unpaid work, are seen as methods through which individuals become members of a variety of communities, in the micro-social sphere, for example.[8]

Obligations and work

The resurrection of debates on obligations as key features of citizenship has been instigated through neo-conservative commentators in the USA and theorists such as Mead (1985), although other ideological traditions are also associated with the idea (Roche 1992: 134-5). This has been accompanied by the growth of 'workfare' policies in the USA (and to a lesser extent in the United Kingdom) whereby recipients of welfare benefits have an obligation to perform work as a corollary of their social 'right' to receive an income from the state. In a perceptive comment on this kind of system, Dahrendorf argues that 'rights are dissolved into marketable commodities; they are offered for sale' (Dahrendorf 1994: 13). The more limited entry of 'workfare' on to the social policy agenda in the United Kingdom has been described by Jessop as an attempt to 'further reduce the drain of unemployment on the exchequer' which he typifies as a measure of short-term political expediency that is symptomatic of 'political drift and economic decay' (Jessop 1994b: 34). Most of the European Left have balked at this kind of imposition of social obligations on welfare recipients, and quite rightly so. The problem is not so much one of obligations and conditions themselves (although there are commentators who advocate complete unconditional universal benefits),[9] but more pertinently the fact that these obligations are imposed only on those who do not possess work for wages. Roche argues that the neo-conservative approach is inherently biased because it does not address the obligations of 'affluent individuals and powerful national and multinational corporations' (Roche 1992: 144). In other words, in a society where the availability of full-time, lifelong work is patently decreasing, it seems odd that only those without work are invested with an obligation to perform socially necessary work. The Left has been rightly wary of a policy which imposes selective work duties on part of the population in a time where work is distributed very unevenly. Thus the notion of universality of rights and obligations is undermined as 'it is the duties of the low-paid, unskilled workers that are the focus of concern, not the higher-paid, skilled and professional workers' (Twine 1994: 165–6). Clearly, this conception of obligation is anathema to the post-industrial socialist project of rethinking and recreating universal citizenship.

Raymond Plant raises other objections to the neo-conservative advocates of 'workfare'. He points out that it is only social rights that are deemed worthy of having these stringent obligations attached to them rather than civil or political rights, which hints at a possible belief among 'workfare' theorists that 'welfare rights are [not] genuine rights at all' (Plant 1993: 44) – a major retreat from universal ideas of citizenship. Moreover, even if we accept the idea of Mead that welfare rights create dependency and irresponsibility among benefit recipients, there is little evidence to suggest that foisting the most meaningless and undesirable work upon them will turn them into shining advertisements of active citizenship. Furthermore, Plant points out that welfare rights are as important as civil rights in providing individuals with security and respect, through, for example, health and education services (Plant 1993: 45). One other criticism put forward by Plant, and it is particularly relevant for the post-industrial Left, is the relationship between duties for work requirements in return for welfare benefits and the state of the labour market as a whole. He points out that any attempt to link welfare rights with work as an obligation must concomitantly involve an economic policy for the state to provide work for welfare claimants to perform. Thus Plant states that:

> It would be inconsistent to insist that work is central to self-respect and that it should be part of the obligation of the citizen if government itself is pursuing policies which actually undermine the very value which is regarded as being at the heart of independent citizenship.
>
> (Plant 1993: 45)

Clearly, very few governments in the world are intent on guaranteeing work for all and, if there was a guarantee of work, there would be little need for social security benefits, although other welfare rights would still have to remain. From the post-industrial socialist perspective, high levels of unemployment and deep social divisions are likely to remain features of advanced capitalist economies, and governments are unlikely to provide work guarantees. This contradiction in governmental policies amounts to what Plant describes as a 'cruel hoax' (Plant 1993: 46). Ultimately, 'workfare' becomes a policy for ensuring that the unemployed perform the most unpleasant work *as and when it is deemed necessary*. This is fundamentally different from an obligation to perform work in return for welfare benefits because work must only be carried out when the state decides that there is some work to be done. This appears to be both cynical and another blow against the principles which underpin universal citizenship. Neo-conservative 'workfare' policies are not designed to make welfare recipients independent individuals acting in the public sphere but, in fact, the opposite. They consign the unemployed to a separate sphere in which the meaningless drudgery which no one else in society wants to perform is carried out, and robs the individuals involved of dignity and self-respect.

Given that the touchstone of post-industrial socialism is the liberation of time and the prioritisation of individual autonomy and collective self-determination, the principle of obligation deployed in 'workfare' is both erroneous and positively harmful. Rather than forging a theory of obligation which involves providing people with fruitful opportunities, the neo-conservative 'workfare' policy is more akin to providing the state with a stick with which to coerce the underprivileged (Jordan 1992: 174). Moreover, 'workfare' emphasises the notion that work in the public sphere is the ultimate activity when that meaningful work is increasingly less available, whereas the post-industrial Left is concerned with the end of work-based society. The inherently workerist notions which substantiate neo-conservative 'workfare' policies are centred upon educating the 'irresponsible' poor into the 'correct' form of behaviour – that is, work for wages – without sufficient work being available for all and, thus, it is difficult not to concur with Roche, who believes that 'it is fanciful, not to say intellectually irresponsible, for Mead and this school of Neo-conservative social analysis to imply that employment *per se* constitutes any kind of serious education for, or even address to, citizenship *per se*' (Roche 1992: 142). The neo-conservative perspective on employment is precisely that which post-industrial socialism is fundamentally opposed to, that is, that only work in the public sphere gives individuals a firm identity and a sense of social citizenship. In this sense I would contend that work for wages provides individuals with a form of social *insertion*, but also that individuals need to find membership of communities and that they require self-identity as autonomous beings. This necessitates a re-evaluation of all activities carried out in the public and private spheres.

Obligations and the post-industrial Left

Given these criticisms of the neo-conservative 'workfare' perspective on obligation, how can the post-industrial Left continue to advocate an obligatory element within their conception of citizenship? If we return to our original thesis that discourses of rights should also encompass theories of duties and remember that post-industrial socialists advocate a right to meaningful work, then we must continue to search for a role for obligations. As Doyal and Gough argue, 'to offer a right to an income with no countervailing obligation to work is ethically dubious, economically debilitating and politically incoherent' (Doyal and Gough 1991: 303). In this sense the inadequacy of current conceptions of obligations of citizenship does not invalidate the claim that social duties are still necessary components of the citizenship equation. The post-industrial Left still has to move beyond the limited obligations to obey the law and pay taxes that are features of liberal democratic citizenship, and the moral authoritarian workerism of neo-conservative advocates of 'workfare'. Turning to the work of André Gorz (as, on the post-industrial Left, he is the clearest writer on social obligations), we can see that his conception of our duties of citizenship is also, at the same time, part of our rights of citizenship (Little 1996: 185–6). In other words, the availability and performance of a limited amount of paid work is viewed as both a right and an obligation on the part of both the individual and the state. Individuals should have a duty to contribute to social wealth by working in the public sphere, while at the same time having a right of access to work in the public sphere. The state has a right to expect everyone who is capable of work in the public sphere to perform a limited amount, while also having an obligation to provide sufficient work for all through a policy of reduced working hours.

The role of the state becomes essential in this scenario for it must facilitate the provision of socially useful work for all and must also develop social policies which can make it feasible for individuals to perform less work for wages. Thus it is incumbent for the state to provide a second income for citizens so that it becomes more desirable to spend less time in work for wages and more in work in the community and autonomous activities. This 'liberation of time' would enable individuals to use their time more fruitfully. It would certainly allow individuals to become more active in communitarian civic activities and provide more time for participation in the politics of whatever communities individuals choose to belong to. In other words, a new politics of time, facilitated by reduced working hours and an obligation to participate in the creation of social wealth, could lead to greater democratic empowerment of the institutions of civil society and communities. Lodziak states that

> the politics of time must proceed hand-in-hand with a politics of
> collective facilities and with a politics of voluntary co-operation
> if the practical expansion of meaningful autonomy for everyone
> is to be realised. If these politics are successful more and more
> people will experience the benefits and satisfactions that ensue
> from activities and projects that they plan, organise and manage
> for themselves.
>
> (Lodziak 1995: 111)

From this it is apparent that the imposition of social obligations for all need not be a threat to autonomy but rather a method of facilitating a social space in which autonomy and collective self-determination could flourish. In this sense, then, the realisation of social interdependence for all people and the embodiment of that interdependence in the performance of socially useful work could open up new spheres of co-operation and freedom outside of the realm of work for wages in the public sphere. If we conclude that the clearest indicator of freedom is the exercise of individual autonomy and participation within chosen collective enterprises in the form of a variety of communities, and that a socialist

approach to liberty and social justice should involve maximal equality of
the resources which provide opportunities to self-determine one's life
choices, then the obligation to perform socially useful work appears to be
a partial step in the trade-off between liberty and equality which post-
industrial socialism involves. Clearly, then, obligations need not be
the exclusionary and divisive tools which they have become in neo-
conservative theory, whereby social and civic responsibility is transplanted
from the state and social institutions to individuals and families without
any concomitant opportunity for individuals to take control over their
lives. According to Gorz, that opportunity can only come about when the
economic right to work is expressed through a thorough reduction of
time spent in work for wages and a new empowerment of individuals and
communities based on the principles of self-determination.

> *Waged* work cannot then continue to be the most important ele-
> ment in our lives . . . they [people] must be given the possibility
> of developing interests and autonomous activities, including
> productive activities. Their socialisation, that is, their insertion
> into society and their sense of belonging to a culture, will derive
> more from these autonomous activities than from the work an
> employer or institution defines for them.
>
> (Gorz 1989a: 231)

This statement makes it clear that post-industrial socialism does not provide a purely economistic perspective on work. It is important that
everyone should have the opportunity to perform work in the public
sphere because the status provided by work is that of being a full
member of society. However, that is only one part of Gorz's equation for
citizenship, which is also concerned with individuals developing
autonomous and collective identities outside the sphere of economic
rationality (i.e. the domain of commodity production and work for
wages). This kind of analysis provides a new dimension in debates over
citizenship which goes beyond the flabby conception of rights in liberal
democracies which could be more accurately described as 'unresourced
opportunities' because they describe formal rights which do not take
into account the ability of individuals to exercise their 'rights'. Moreover,
the post-industrial Left is keen to concretise a theory of obligation which
reciprocates the theory of rights, although this does not have to be
understood in a purely direct manner. This involves providing individuals with tangible duties to others and the state which enshrine socialist
citizenship, and also regulating the state to ensure that it provides both
the opportunities and resources whereby autonomous individuals can

experience their citizenship. Within this theoretical framework we can begin to examine policy proposals which incorporate post-industrial socialist values. First, however, we must examine theories of human need which become central when the aim is a total overhaul of welfare provision and, from there, we can measure the extent to which radical social policy alternatives meet theoretical perspectives on need, and simultaneously fulfil the criteria for citizenship outlined by the post-industrial Left. Thus, in the words of Offe, we must seek a regeneration of welfare provision which 'emphasize[s] the values of security *and* autonomy, and envisage the possibility of reconciling the alleged antagonism between the two in relying upon the idea of *citizenship* and the positive rights and entitlements . . . associated with it' (Offe 1992: 70). There is, however, another dimension to the reappraisal of state welfare about which the post-industrial Left has not been quite so forthright – the notion of human needs.

4

LEFT-LIBERTARIANISM, AUTONOMY AND HUMAN NEEDS

One of the most controversial areas in contemporary welfare debates concerns theories of human needs. Part of the reason for the contested nature of this area comes in the problem of defining human needs in an *ex ante* manner when our perceptions of what needs actually are may, by their nature, be *ex post* due to the social context in which they are formulated. The tendency of the post-industrial Left has been to focus on this distortion of perceptions of human needs in advanced capitalist societies (which has been exacerbated by the growth of consumerism). While this is a central aspect of explaining the dynamics of industrial societies, a Left-libertarian viewpoint on human needs is an essential part of constructing a fitting welfare theory for post-industrial socialism. However, a clear outline of a theory of human needs has not been forthcoming to date from the post-industrial Left. In an attempt to clarify this situation this chapter will begin with an analysis of Left-libertarian social theory on the manipulation of needs under capitalism with particular regard to the work of Conrad Lodziak (1986, 1995), who has been forthright in constructing a position which owes much to critical theory. From this basis we can then move on to evaluate the most developed theory of human need that has been articulated in recent years, that of Len Doyal and Ian Gough (1991). Finally, we can set out criteria for post-industrial socialist welfare theory by combining the previous examination of needs theories with a discussion of rights. This will provide a foundation for an analysis of potential policy proposals for the post-industrial Left in the closing chapters of the book.

The manipulation of needs

A characteristic of Leftist positions on human needs from Marx to contemporary Left-libertarians has been the problematic nature of their identification given the manipulation of their meaning within capitalism. What once were perceived as wants and luxuries in previous eras come to be seen as necessities in subsequent times. However, the fact that this is the case does not and should not in itself invalidate attempts to formulate such a theory on which to base models of social welfare. This is not to say that in practice these models and theories are perfectible but that they provide the guidelines through which developments in social welfare can be measured and gauged. Before developing a theory of human needs, however, it is important to understand the ways in which needs are manipulated in advanced capitalism as a post-industrial socialist society which promotes self-limitation would clearly be based upon non-consumerist and anti-materialist foundations. The rejection of consumerism and materialism suggests that the prevalence of these values within advanced capitalism generates false needs which are actually no more than desires. The Left-libertarian perspective on true and false needs was articulated by Marcuse, who suggested that emancipation had to be derived from a rejection of the rationality that was transmitted by capitalist institutions.

> [E]conomic freedom would mean freedom *from* the economy – from being controlled by economic forces and relationships; freedom from the daily struggle for existence, from earning a living. Political freedom would mean liberation of the individuals *from* politics over which they have no effective control . . . The most effective and enduring form of warfare against liberation is the implanting of material and intellectual needs that perpetuate obsolete forms of the struggle for existence.
>
> (Marcuse 1986: 4)

Although this identifies with the emancipatory aims of post-industrial socialism insofar as it is founded on the notion of rejecting the rationality of industrial capitalism and recognises that human needs are historical in their character, it does not make the task of formulating a theory (however transient) any less important. In other words the satisfaction of needs will invariably change as societies develop, but this does not mean that there are not broad and basic categories of human need, it merely recognises that there will be variations in modes of need satisfaction.

The aim for Marcuse was to articulate the primacy of autonomy as a goal for the Left as he believed that it was only really autonomous individuals that were able to experience and satisfy their own needs. In this sense individual needs as we understand them under advanced capitalism involve emancipation from the goals and values of that rationality which distorts our perceptions of our needs. Liberation, then, becomes a human need because the 'distinguishing feature of advanced industrial society is its effective suffocation of those needs which demand liberation . . . while it sustains and absolves the destructive power and repressive function of the affluent society' (Marcuse 1986: 7). Thus Marcuse's position was one where capitalism, through the repression of individual autonomy, generates 'false' needs which can only be genuinely distinguished from 'true' needs if individuals are liberated from the logic of industrialisation. He recognised, of course, that there are basic needs such as food, clothing and shelter but also that the satisfaction of these most basic of needs is the only form of need satisfaction which can be discerned and defended in advanced capitalism, as they are biologically determined. All other emotions and feelings are generated in an historical condition characterised by the absence of freedom, and are therefore inadmissible as human needs.

Marcuse's approach is valuable because it centres on the ways in which needs are manipulated by the socio-economic conditions in which they are experienced, yet they suggest such is the power and prevalence of the rationality and ideology of industrialism that attempts to outline a different theory of needs governed by a non-economic rationality will ultimately founder. However, there is a glimmer of hope in Marcuse's position insofar as he argued that the internalisation of the needs that are generated in advanced capitalism and the inability of society to meet those needs may lead to the necessary qualitative changes which would further his goal of human liberation. Thus he clearly points out that this involves a 'redefinition of needs' (Marcuse 1986: 245). Taking this perspective on board, it can be argued that post-industrial socialism provides a significant political impetus in developing an alternative philosophy on which to build a qualitative redefinition of needs, based as it is upon the inversion of capitalist economic rationality and a new politics of time. Such an enterprise has been developed by Lodziak (1995: 70–2), who has employed the ideas of Marcuse and Habermas in outlining what he refers to as the manipulation of needs thesis. This involves four key interacting characteristics:

- The capitalist system controls the resources which individuals have at their disposal to satisfy their needs.
- The capitalist system manipulates time which individuals might spend pursuing autonomous activities.
- The dynamic of the reproduction of the capitalist system is provided by the restriction of individual autonomy.

- The capitalist system provides only privatistic and meaningless opportunities to develop identities, which reinforces the reproduction of the system.

For Lodziak the outcome of this process is the idea that

> a significant proportion of the population do not experience the multitude of choices that are available as sufficiently meaningful and satisfying. In other words whatever the attractions of consumerism, and our new found freedoms, they fail to satisfy what the individual needs to sustain a meaningful sense of self.
>
> (Lodziak 1995: 20)

This corresponds with some of the gloomier points that Marcuse put forward in *One-dimensional Man* but the book also contained a more optimistic strand which identifies how the reproductive, self-referential system can be overcome if a new oppositional culture is built around the idea of a new politics of time. In this sense the arguments which Lodziak develops provide a Left-libertarian theoretical backdrop to the formation of a post-industrial socialist politics. Where Marcuse was rather tentative about the possibilities of emerging from the embrace of industrial society and the perpetuating logic of consumerism, Lodziak is able to identify more fruitful ground for organising opposition to the dominant ideology (although he is very well aware of the institutionalised obstacles and barriers that prevent popular mobilisation against capitalist reproduction). Thus we can identify a Left-libertarian theory which suggests that advanced capitalism generates false needs which negate themselves insofar as they are unable to generate self-identity, and therefore a potentially emancipatory process is in place because identity needs remain unsatisfied. To date, advanced capitalism has managed to reproduce continually because the unsatisfied needs are replaced by other 'false' needs, not least because the dynamic of society is still an economic rationality which pervades all areas of social existence. It is the opposition to that very rationality which contains the potential for post-industrial socialism and the development of 'a culture of opposition' (Lodziak 1995).

However, before moving on to an outline of human needs as part of a philosophy of emancipation, it is important to understand the extent of the manipulation of needs that is suggested by commentators such as Lodziak. On the social level the manipulation of needs thesis rests upon the contraction of the public sphere and the erosion of civic values therein. These values, which are beneficial to the formation of self-identity, are manipulated and manufactured by the overarching logic of economic values of growth and profit. On the individual level this process is reflected by the growth of privatistic motivation in constructing self-identity which is often equated (not always correctly) with the expansion of individualism at the expense of the common interest. According to Lodziak, this individualistic ethos, often manifest in consumerism, is presented as freedom when in effect it only represents an inappropriate and ineffective means of satisfying identity needs. Against the claims of theorists such as Bauman (1992), Lodziak suggests that:

> Basic identity needs, such as a sense of security and a sense of significance, relate more to the development and maintenance of meaningful and satisfying identities than to the continual symbolic construction and reconstruction of identities . . . This is not to deny that consumer goods are of symbolic value – they most certainly are. But what I am saying is that the symbolic is largely irrelevant to identity needs . . . If our identities are tied to consumerism, they will always be in transition and thus destabilised and unsatisfying.
>
> (Lodziak 1995: 50)

This has serious implications for a philosophy which analyses the theory of human needs in terms of self-identity and the effects of modern life on identity formation. Lodziak believes that regardless of what identities we develop (or could develop under different social organisation), they must be stable and capable of providing some permanency in self-worth and security. In other words, Lodziak's conception of identity needs equates to stability and ontological security. It is from this basis that individuals can develop autonomously to enjoy their freedom. Giddens refers to these kinds of ideas when he suggests that emancipatory politics is based upon the principle of autonomy in which: 'Freedom presumes acting responsibly in relation to others and recognising that collective obligations are involved' (Giddens 1991: 213). It is this principle which is rarely exercised in advanced capitalism due to the organisation of time and resources. For Lodziak, most of us are in one way or another dependent on paid work (either through working ourselves, being dependent on others who work, or being available for work in order to receive welfare benefits) to gain resources to enable us to act upon our limited preferences in the time left over from work. This dependency mitigates against our opportunities to make autonomous choices about our actions and leaves us with very limited spheres of action: 'The choices available to people are restricted by the resources that are available. This means that in explaining action we must, first and foremost, take account of the resources that are available *and not available*' (Lodziak 1995: 56). What then are the implications of this dependency in terms of individualism and privatism and what effects do these phenomena have on our interpretation of individual autonomy?

In answering this question Lodziak distinguishes between 'survival' and 'beyond survival' or 'existential' needs such as ontological security.[1] Where, according to Marcuse, survival needs are broadly accepted (although the attacks on the British welfare state in the 1980s might suggest the opposite at least in terms of who is responsible for need satisfaction), 'beyond survival' needs are more contentious. This situation provides the impetus behind Lodziak's conception of the need for autonomy:

> There are universal needs beyond survival. What people seek is a meaningful and satisfying life. But what is meaningful and satisfying cannot be prescribed for us. What is meaningful and satisfying for one person may not be so for another . . . [T]he surest way this need can be met is for individuals to control their own lives. In other words the need for a meaningful and satisfying life translates into the need for autonomy.
>
> (Lodziak 1995: 62)

However, the experience of advanced capitalism is one where autonomy – and the need for it – has been surrendered and has been theoretically appropriated by a notion of individual freedom which finds its apogee in consumerism. Lodziak is quick to point to the ideological nature of this type of individualism. It is something people do, not something which most people are actually committed to or motivated by. Indeed, he argues that such is the transient and ephemeral nature of consumerism that the experience is not something that people use to satisfy identity needs except on the most ostensible level. Why, then, is consumerism so rampant? The answer to this, according to Lodziak, is the phenomenon of privatism which encompasses a cultural trend involving 'social and political withdrawal or abstinence, and coupled with this a central focus on family and domestic life, and/or some form of self-absorption' (Lodziak 1995: 75). Where current social trends are often depicted as a by-product of the growth of individualism (and an ideological commitment to self-interest), Lodziak sees this process as a situation in which people are coerced into attempting to satisfy identity needs in the private sphere through the dearth of opportunities that are available for identity formation in the public domain. However, privatism is not described as a unitary phenomenon but one which takes several different but overlapping forms which have been discussed extensively by Habermas (1976), Williams (1983) and Lodziak (1986) in demonstrating that it is not merely a manifestation of an individualist ethos.[2] Essentially, Lodziak (1995: 75–6) identifies three main forms of privatism:

- mobile privatism – this equates to the private consumption of goods and services in relation to the family and domestic life;
- self-maintaining privatism – the consumption of goods on the basis of satisfying survival needs;
- post-necessity privatism – this equates to a limited form of self-actualisation.

These three forms of privatism do overlap with each other as motivation for action varies, but Lodziak's key argument is that none of them equates to a total ideological commitment to or incorporation by individualist rationality. Certainly, within advanced capitalism these phenomena help to reproduce the dominant form of social organisation, but the activities, in themselves, are not inherently individualistic in motivation. Indeed, the failure of privatism with regard to the satisfaction of 'beyond survival' needs provides a foundational point in Lodziak's advocacy of an oppositional culture. This culture cannot derive its basis within privatism (as this helps to reinforce the dominant system and is self-perpetuating) but privatism can be halted if we recognise its inadequacy in providing autonomy. Moreover, the prevalence of privatism suggests that individuals are seeking avenues for self-actualisation and the satisfaction of self-identity needs. Therefore, Lodziak argues that 'the expansion of that sphere of autonomy embraces the traditional and more contemporary concerns of emancipatory politics, and is thus an appropriate unifying focus for oppositional politics' (Lodziak 1995: 117). In this sense we need to formulate a firmer definition of identity needs and identify the place that they have in recent debates on broader theories of human need (Doyal and Gough 1991; Gough 1993; Soper 1993)

A theory of human needs

The orthodox Marxist position on needs, which is usually associated with the principle contained in *Critique of the Gotha Programme* of 'From each according to his ability, to each according to his needs', has been criticised in more recent times due to the fragmentation of the working class. Thus G. A. Cohen has argued that a problem arises in Marxist thinking when a separation occurs between those who are directly exploited by capitalists (the working class) and the 'needy people in society' who are, in contemporary times, often not working (Cohen 1995: 155; Kymlicka 1990: 193–4) – for Cohen, the fact that these people might be exploited in other ways is irrelevant (Cohen 1995: 155) For the post-industrial Left, of course, such a condition is not irrelevant because it is based on the lived experience of the oppressed in advanced capitalism rather than an imaginary philosophical subject. However, Cohen is correct to identify that no one group holds the requisite features of Marx's proletariat that would bring about revolution. Thus a philosophy of social change that is based on a coherent theory of human need cannot *solely* be based upon the needs of the least well-off, although, of course, they are the most likely to encounter the absence of need satisfaction. In other words, the decline of the theoretical unified exploited class as an historical agent to be overtaken by a variety of groups who face broader oppression which can take a range of different forms *necessitates* a theory of human need which is broadly applicable and not just focused on the most exploited.[3] Where Cohen argues that the Marxian need principle is relegated in importance when need and exploitation become detached, the post-industrial Left believes that this actually accentuates the importance of a theory of human need. This is especially true when such a theory is not just predicated on survival needs alone but is broadened to encompass existential and identity needs. The non-satisfaction of identity needs can afflict anyone whether their survival needs are met or not (although, again, it should be easier to meet identity needs if one's survival needs have already been met).

The theory of needs which best fits Left-libertarian principles is one where broad generic categories of need are identified, including both 'survival' and 'beyond survival' needs, but also one in which the method of satisfaction of those needs will vary between different individuals and social and cultural groups. This chapter is therefore concerned with identifying needs, not prescribing how individuals should satisfy them. The latter will vary not least because of changing social conditions and the different identities that individuals formulate. In the words of Doyal and Gough:

> Human needs ... are neither subjective preferences best understood by each individual, nor static essences best understood by planners or party officials. They are universal and knowable, but our knowledge of them, and of the satisfiers necessary to meet them, is dynamic and open-ended.
>
> (Doyal and Gough 1991: 4)

Perspectives on human needs

Doyal and Gough have provided the most thorough conceptualisation of human need in recent years.[4] Their work provides a rigorous defence of why human needs must be theorised, a sophisticated and well-formulated theory of need, a comparative recognition of what need satisfaction might mean in practice, and the strategic political implications of their theoretical proposition. Initially, they set out six different perspectives on the notion of human needs (Doyal and Gough 1991: chs 1 and 2):

- orthodox economics;
- the New Right;
- Marxism;
- critiques of cultural imperialism;
- radical democrats;
- phenomenological arguments.

The orthodox economics approach views action almost solely in terms of economic activity. In this scenario individuals are consumers and the expression of their preferences through what they consume is a reflection of their needs. This approach tends to conflate wants and needs, and prioritises the role of individuals in deciding their own interests. In this perspective human need cannot be objectively defined but, as Doyal and Gough argue, this view suffers once we understand that individuals cannot have a full grasp of the possibilities for rational action (Hutton 1996) and, therefore, the welfare that will derive from each activity cannot be accurately weighed up. In this sense orthodox economics falls into the very trap that Left-libertarians warn against – it wrongly equates wants expressed through economic behaviour with needs. The second main perspective, that of the New Right, derives impetus from classical economics insofar as it agrees that individual preferences are superior to those decided by the state and as such liberalised markets are the arenas where needs should be met because they are the most efficient means of distribution. However, the New Right 'are not morally neutral about capitalism. They believe that it is a good thing – that the productivity and freedom which they claim it engenders is worth encouraging and defending' (Doyal and Gough 1991: 25). Thus, like the orthodox economics approach, the New Right resorts to the essentialisation of 'the market'. Moreover, there is the perennial problem with the utility of market mechanisms which is that the outcomes of their operation presupposes that everyone who enters into them has the same chance of success in meeting their preferential needs – in other words, they do not recognise that some people have more chance of satisfying their wants in markets than others. For post-industrial socialism, both orthodox economists and the New Right make the mistake of equating need satisfaction with the workings of market mechanisms. Certainly, markets have a role to play in post-industrial politics but they have very little to do with the satisfaction or even recognition of human needs (Gorz 1988). The point here is that there are some spheres where market mechanisms and rationality are appropriate and others where they are not. This type of theory is hinted at by Hahn, who argues that 'citizens might have utilitarian norms in one subspace or for certain neighbourhoods in that space without being utilitarian *tout court*' (Hahn 1996: 15).

The third perspective which Doyal and Gough identify is the Marxist approach to human needs. They relate the Marxist position, which corresponds with that of Marcuse above, as follows: 'the economic aspects of the social environment were by far the most important in shaping human identity' (Doyal and Gough 1991: 12). However, as with Marcuse, there appears to be a potential lifeline in Marxist thought on human needs:

> Marx thought that the social relations of capitalism are uniquely constituted to lead to a veritable explosion in human productivity and material expectation, bringing in their train a 'constantly enriched system of needs'. These new needs are not only testimony to the creativity of the human spirit. In the midst of large-scale poverty and exploitation, they also sow the seeds of revolt through underlining what might be – the prospect of abundance and the injustice of a social system where the needs of those who produce the wealth remain unmet.
>
> (Doyal and Gough 1991: 13)

The upshot of this position leaves potential for more thorough perspectives of human needs to develop in capitalist societies but at the same time we should be clear that Marx saw genuine understanding of needs as a by-product of the undermining of the economic base of capitalist society. Doyal and Gough note the contradictions in the orthodox Marxist position insofar as to deny all conceptions of human need *until* capitalism has been overcome makes it highly difficult actually to ascertain *when* capitalism has been overcome. In other words, without an available conception of human needs it is difficult to identify which needs are not met within advanced capitalism and which would be met in whatever model of post-capitalist society one adheres to. Thus, without a thorough conception of human needs, Marxism looks overly determinist in relation to the economy and not developed enough in providing a strategic alternative to advanced capitalism. Moreover, Doyal and Gough note that pressing ecological problems of the contemporary world suggest that a new Leftist theory of needs cannot rest on abundance of resources as in orthodox Marxism, but rather must involve placing needs within the context of scarce resources (Doyal and Gough 1991). This is what Gorz refers to when he suggests that self-limitation is a central concept in the regeneration of radical theories of need: 'Political ecology . . . uses ecologically *necessary* changes to the mode of production and consumption as a lever for normatively *desirable* changes in the mode of life and in social relations' (Gorz 1993: 65).

The fourth perspective on need which Doyal and Gough identify is that of the critiques of cultural imperialism which suggest that needs cannot be prescribed by one group for another. From this approach *universal* needs are not applicable, not least because some groups have considerably more power than others which could be reflected in the conception of need that is developed. The most obvious strands of this stream of thought identified by Doyal and Gough come from anti-racists and feminists who, despite the similarities in their general critiques, also have fundamental differences when it comes to human needs.[5] This poses a particularly stringent question for advocates of universal needs, especially in light of the fact that their proposals are designed to incorporate the needs of the most oppressed, which includes, by their own claims, women and ethnic minorities. However, the *existence* of needs is not at issue, rather the opponents of cultural imperialism object to the creation of a taxonomy of needs by people who have not faced the same oppression as those who have been subject to that oppression. Doyal and Gough criticise this approach on the grounds that universalism becomes redundant when the rights of any group to do what it likes become paramount. Where pluralism is to be encouraged to the greatest possible extent, the notion that we cannot submit what we deem to be unpleasant activities to criticism appears to turn pluralism on its head. Again the central principle for needs theory should be the identification of broad universal human needs which can be satisfied in a range of particularistic and pluralistic fashions. This stance will not meet all of the challenges that are likely to arise in contemporary societies (and one could argue nor should it) but it should go some way to developing a more satisfactory and tolerant framework in which disputes can be mediated.[6]

Doyal and Gough believe that the points of the critiques of cultural imperialism have particular resonance when directed at the proponents of their fifth approach, the radical democrats who see needs as discursive. This category is applied to moderate pluralists such as Michael Walzer (1983) and more radical proponents of a pluralist socialism such as

Laclau and Mouffe (1985) and others who can be attached to the post-industrial Left such as Keane (1988).[7] Doyal and Gough argue that these commentators pay insufficient attention to the role of the state as the guarantor of human needs, preferring instead to promote the under-standing of needs within the context of civil society. However, the commentators themselves are a touch more varied than Doyal and Gough would have us believe. Walzer perhaps is a fair victim of their cri-tique, although there is a highly persuasive dimension to his defence of pluralism in civil society. Keane (and Laclau and Mouffe) on the other hand are much more reserved in their promotion of civil society in the sense that they understand that there must be a strong role for the state in providing the appropriate conditions under which the institutions of civil society are able to flourish. Keane is very clear that this process will be facilitated in negotiation with the state or it will not happen. That said, Doyal and Gough are wise to counsel that public regulation of the work-ings of civil society is necessary:

> [W]ithout a coherent theory of human need to inform such regulation – especially in the context of capitalism and the dis-torted perceptions of need which follow from it – there is little choice but to lapse into an optimistic and hazardous idealism that, when left alone, individuals and groups will always know what is best for them . . . They won't and they don't.
>
> (Doyal and Gough 1991: 31)

Of course, they are reasonable in suggesting that we need to be careful about the sidetracking of the issues of human needs into a relativist sphere of civil society, but this does not mean that we should abandon the sphere of civil society as a vital domain in which needs can be satisfied. Yet again, the clear delineation of universal human needs and particu-laristic notions of need satisfaction is relevant here, especially if we view the state as the defender of universalism with regard to needs, and groups within civil society as the media through which needs can be experienced and satisfied in contingent circumstances. In this sense, Hewitt argues that Doyal and Gough have provided a theory of 'univer-sal needs that different cultural communities or social movements seek to satisfy, whether by productive labour or social struggle. The point is that it is possible cogently to articulate a set of links between the universal and particular dimensions of need' (Hewitt 1996: 212; see also Jones 1990: 39–40; Spicker 1993/4).

The final perspective on needs which Doyal and Gough address emanates from phenomenological sociology which holds that perceptions of need tend to be socially constructed and that no objective categorisation of needs is possible as they are essentially subjective. While this perspective should not be disregarded because it ascribes vast importance to individual perceptions (which are valuable in the sense that they are lived experiences), it does not focus enough on the distortion of those perceptions in advanced capitalism. Again this leans too close to cultural relativism for Doyal and Gough, who are quick to note how relativists tend to be inconsistent: for example, insofar as they will tend to use universalism when it suits the ideological purposes which they hope it will serve. Moreover, 'the consistent relativist – one who regards the whole of social life as a "construction", each aspect of which has no more or less veracity then any other – enters a moral wasteland into which few have feared to tread' (Doyal and Gough 1991: 33).

The theory of human needs and post-industrial socialism

For the post-industrial Left, the resonance of the Doyal and Gough thesis is clear enough. The critique of orthodox and welfare economics and the New Right rejection of needs-based theory fits comfortably with Left-libertarian philosophy. Economically determinist Marxism is also problematic, although in criticising determinism we must be careful to acknowledge that even if the economic system does not determine social relations, it does influence the ways in which we understand our needs and thus the strategies we might pursue to satisfy them. Similarly, we must recognise that, despite the weaknesses that Doyal and Gough identify, there is some veracity in the claims of opponents of cultural imperialism and phenomenological arguments over social construction. It is only by addressing the needs which are ascribed to various groups that we can establish whether they are truly particular needs or whether they are actually just different forms of need satisfaction which do not practically undermine the principle of universalism. This is where the radical democratic approach which Doyal and Gough identify also has utility for the post-industrial Left. In outlining how a radically different polity in which communities and intermediate institutions were empowered within the sphere of civil society could be to the benefit of a range of groups, radical democrats are providing a framework through which variegated need satisfaction could take place within the institutions of civil society while the state would guarantee that universal needs would be satisfied. The point that deserves to be reiterated is that the state must act as a mediator between different bodies, institutions and communities and as a guarantor of universalism, but that the means of satisfying needs will vary between different individuals and communities. In no sense, then, are radical democrats or post-industrial socialists dismissive of the role of the state as the facilitator of the conditions to allow the non-state sector to work adequately.[8] In the words of John Keane:

> [A] democratic civil society could never go it alone . . . it requires state power actively to defend its independence. Democratisation is neither the outright enemy nor the unconditional friend of state power. It requires the state to govern civil society neither too much [n]or too little; while a more democratic order cannot be built *through* state power, it cannot be built *without* state power.
>
> (Keane 1988: 23)

This point is vital. Post-industrial socialism concurs with the radical democrat approach that the state has a key role to play in provision for human needs, not just in terms of actually providing the services themselves but in devolving the ability to satisfy needs to individuals, communities, trade unions and other co-operative groups from religious bodies to self-help groups. This is not a utopian philosophy of harmonious social relations but rather a recognition of conflict and disagreement that might arise between groups. The point is that the resolution of conflict (over needs or a variety of other issues) is more likely to come about if all parties are empowered and tolerant of difference which is the process which the state must facilitate.

In the second part of their book Doyal and Gough justify their critique of the other approaches by outlining their own theory of human needs. Essentially they identify two key principles which provide the impetus for creating such a theory: participation and liberation. Indeed, they also suggest that provision to allow opportunities for participation actually contributes to the goal of liberation. This corresponds with post-industrial socialist ideas about the importance of social contribution in the formation of self-identity and maintenance of ontological security. Thus, 'unless individuals are capable of participating in some form of life without arbitrary and serious limitations being placed on what they attempt to accomplish, their potential for private and public success will remain unfulfilled – whatever the detail of their actual choices' (Doyal and Gough 1991: 50). This entails a range of factors, not least the absence of serious harm, which involves a basic need for both physical health and autonomy of agency. In turn these basic needs are predicated upon the satisfaction of a range of intermediate needs which Doyal and Gough (1991: 157–8) define as:

- nutritional food and clean water;
- protective housing;
- a non-hazardous work environment;
- a non-hazardous physical environment;
- appropriate health care;
- security in childhood;
- significant primary relationships;
- physical security;
- economic security;
- appropriate education;
- safe birth control and child-bearing.

These criteria are designed to provide a theory of need which transcends the divisions and specific needs of a range of groups. Moreover, they recognise that the satisfaction (or not) of some of these intermediate needs overlap with or contribute to each other. Thus those that we can identify as survival needs definitely contribute to the conditions under which 'beyond survival' needs can be met. The satisfaction of 'beyond survival' needs such as significant relationships or security is accomplished more easily if our needs for shelter or food have already been satisfied and do not require constant attention. It should also be noted that the nature of the definition of intermediate needs in Doyal and Gough's theory makes them widely applicable and resilient to relativism. For example, the suggestion that we have a need for 'protective housing' does not prescribe what type of housing people in a specific geographical location require – obviously this will vary (as will the cost of that housing). Similarly, the proposal that individuals need autonomy of agency to acquire a degree of social participation does not entail the idea that everyone will experience or use their autonomy in the same ways.

Doyal and Gough go back one more degree in outlining societal preconditions which would adequately enable individuals to satisfy their needs in a self-determined manner. They argue that their promotion of autonomy is not an individualist philosophy in the sense that, unless social organisation is properly defined, autonomy will not be experienced in a universal fashion. In this sense Doyal and Gough state that

> the opportunity to express individual autonomy requires much more than simply being left alone – more than negative freedom. If we really were ignored by others, we never learn the rules of our way of life and thereby acquire the capacity to make choices within it ... In other words, to be autonomous and to be physically healthy, we also require *positive freedom* – material,

> educational and emotional need satisfaction . . . Against the
> background of the general socialisation on which their cognitive
> and emotional capacity for action depends, autonomous indi-
> viduals (who are not slaves) must understand why they should
> not physically constrain the actions of others and must possess
> the emotional competence to act accordingly.
>
> (Doyal and Gough 1991: 78–9)

Again this perspective corresponds with the Left-libertarian philosophy which post-industrial socialism embodies. In this sense we can only under-stand our individual freedoms within the context of the society and communities of which we are a part and the freedoms of the other indi-viduals within those entities. This has particular resonance when it comes to the advocacy of 'the end of work-based society' because the latter depends upon the equitable distribution of socially necessary work for three main reasons. First, work in the public sphere is seen as a primary form of social participation and contribution, and should, therefore, be something which we understand as a human need. Second, if we view this process as a human need and we are attempting to formulate a means through which human needs can be satisfied, then work needs to be more equitably distributed, which will involve reduced working hours so that everyone is provided with more opportunities to engage in mean-ingful work. Third, because work is not the only means of achieving social identity, it is in the interests of the development of individual autonomy to limit the number of hours spent in work for wages so that individuals can pursue other activities which are either self-determined or necessary but unpaid. In this sense the need for autonomy coupled with the principle of positive liberty involves an obligation for individuals to limit working hours which can only be achieved through widespread negotiation and planning on the state level and in more localised domains.

Taking needs theory to thorough conclusions, then, we have to envis-age the social organisation which will allow us to understand the main features of need satisfaction. The four universal societal preconditions for need satisfaction which Doyal and Gough identify are:

1   the process of *production* which relates to the social relations of pro-duction and the economic system of any given society;
2   biological *reproduction* and socialisation (the forms of which may vary between different societies);
3   *cultural transmission* which refers to the process of reproducing social structures;

4   *authority* which the authors use to refer to a state which will hold the power of sanctions to protect accepted social structures.

These criteria are the fundamental building blocks of society in the Doyal and Gough thesis to the extent that they 'refer to the structural activities which any minimally successful mode of social life must be able to carry out. They also refer to concrete goals whose achievement must be planned for and sustained over time' (Doyal and Gough 1991: 89).

While these features are not particularly controversial, there are some environmental constraints which post-industrial socialists might refer to in this area. First, the focus on *material* production in the Doyal and Gough thesis needs to be couched in the terms of scarcity and therefore the notion that material production as it exists can be sustained must be reassessed alongside the promotion of self-limitation which corresponds with post-materialist concerns with limits to economic growth.[9] Similarly, some recognition of environmental constraints on population growth would strengthen the contemporary and future applicability of Doyal and Gough's ideas on reproduction (although it should be noted that they are as concerned with birth control as reproduction itself). The third criterion they identify, cultural transmission, is clearly central to social reproduction, although the post-industrial Left would be concerned with clearer opportunities for the promotion of an oppositional culture in which a dominant ideology of capitalist reproduction such as economic rationality could be challenged. Finally, post-industrial socialists such as Gorz and radical democrats like Keane are clearly advocates of a strong role for the state in establishing political authority but, more explicitly than Doyal and Gough, they are also very concerned with widespread devolution of power and authority to intermediate institutions such as community groups in civil society and trade unions in the workplace.

The other dimension of the Doyal and Gough thesis which should be developed here is the primary role of 'critical autonomy' in their perception of the achievement of participation and liberation. Initially, it is useful to outline that the list of intermediate needs above is deemed to be essential in the development of individual autonomy. In this sense individuals cannot be genuinely autonomous with respect to having power to act upon their choices if they have not already satisfied their survival needs. The choices available to an individual may be severely restrained if they cannot afford to feed themselves (and their children) or find decent housing. However, at the same time it is, of course, possible that individuals can have their survival needs satisfied and not experience full autonomy. Indeed, this is the crux of the thesis constructed by Left-libertarians such as Marcuse and Lodziak insofar as individual self-identity needs are deemed to be predominantly unsatisfied despite continued existence and social reproduction. This is why a radical theory of human needs which centres upon the qualitative experience of life must deal with the issue of 'beyond survival' needs in which autonomy is the central principle. For Doyal and Gough:

> Three key variables affect levels of individual autonomy: the level of *understanding* a person has about herself, her culture and what is expected of her as an individual within it; the *psychological capacity* she has to formulate options for herself; and the objective *opportunities* enabling her to act accordingly.
>
> (Doyal and Gough 1991: 60)

However, even this degree of autonomy as agency is not sufficient for Doyal and Gough. They correctly note that these conditions could be met within a range of regimes in which key freedoms are repressed, such as under totalitarianism. Their preferred form of autonomy is what they term 'critical autonomy', in which individuals not only have the ability to make choices but also the capacity and *power* to influence those choices. Thus where 'the opportunity exists to question and to participate in agreeing or changing the rules of a culture, it will be possible for actors significantly to increase their autonomy through a spectrum of choices unavailable to the politically oppressed . . . what was autonomy becomes "critical autonomy" ' (Doyal and Gough 1991: 67). The point here is that the ability to make political choices and to participate in the political process (in the broadest sense of this notion) amounts to a higher level of autonomy than autonomy of agency. Moreover, Doyal and Gough believe that individuals who have 'critical autonomy' are more likely to be critical in their participation in social life.[10] This is a central point for the post-industrial Left as it opens up opportunities whereby individuals, provided with greater choice of activities than work-for-wages, may react against the economic rationality and ideology of work which currently permeates the public sphere. In the words of Eriksen:

> The stability and durability of democracy and the rationality of collective decision making are interdependent. The unequal distribution of goods and commodities decreases the quality of the citizenship as fewer are able to participate on equal terms in the public deliberation of what to do . . . To provide individuals with goods and commodities in order to make them active citizens . . . can be justified as a collective goal.
>
> (Eriksen 1996: 63)

The final point to note in this section has direct relevance to the issue raised above and the general position of the post-industrial left on welfare. Doyal and Gough propose that in terms of meeting needs in markets there should be a right to a minimum income attached to a rationally and democratically agreed level which would be sufficient to meet basic needs.[11] They are somewhat tentative on this issue in pointing briefly to two possible options, a basic income scheme or a policy of guaranteed full employment, but simultaneously noting problems with both. As we shall see in the final chapters of this book, neither of these options really fits adequately with post-industrial socialist theory, but a fusion of the two might come closer to the ideal. In any case this is where we reach the nub of the argument in identifying potential policy alternatives for the post-industrial Left. Before moving on to that territory, however, it is necessary to conclude this chapter with an examination of the relationship between human needs and rights to need satisfaction through welfare.

Needs, rights and welfare

Given the inefficiencies of the welfare state that post-industrial socialists highlight, it is important to identify why they continue to advocate such a central role for the state in providing the conditions under which social welfare will flourish. In other words, it is necessary to understand how the needs that individuals experience are to be satisfied in political practice and thus how *some* human needs can be translated into social rights. This involves analysis of which needs can be translated into the discourse of rights and thus of how needs come to play a central role in the achievement of social justice (N. Barry 1992: 49). For the post-industrial Left this issue involves the notion that our perception of needs should be understood in terms of creating the conditions under which their satisfaction, especially when it comes to 'beyond survival' needs, is seen as a positive phenomenon and not merely as a negative situation in which we only see their satisfaction as the avoidance of harm (Spicker 1993: 7). In this sense human needs (and their satisfaction) are not to be understood in a purely mechanical sense in which their satisfaction is measurable, but as general categories in which quality of life is assessed. For instance, even the need for adequate shelter or food is an area where the notion of adequacy is open to empirical dispute, but this does not negate the necessity of shelter. Thus the Left-libertarian philosophy that we assess our need satisfaction on the basis of our having the autonomous capability to do so becomes the operative principle. Eriksen states that: 'Claims of need satisfaction can . . . no longer be justified by invoking *one* concept of the good society but have to appeal to universal interests, that is, something that can be made valid across cultural differences and shifting notions of the good life' (Eriksen 1996: 68). The choices of autonomous individuals then supersede the decisions of need made by professionals according to strictly defined 'objective' criteria. The latter perspective equates with the view expounded by Spicker, who sees needs not as human phenomena but as competing claims on available resources (Spicker 1993: 7). The post-industrial socialist perspective contends that needs are not claims on material resources but instead the experience of individuals having the capacity to take control over need satisfaction themselves. Undoubtedly, as we shall see, this involves individuals having the resources to take control over decision-making. In this sense social rights then become the rights to the resources which facilitate individual need satisfaction. This does not invalidate the principle of need or the necessity of the state providing certain services to assist the opportunities open to autonomous individuals. Thus,

> rights are not propensities which vest naturally in every individual but represent specific demands or claims for resources and/or services. Certainly, a need becomes a right when it is formulated as a claim; but there is a sense in which needs, rights and claims are all expressions of human dependence.
>
> (Dean 1996: 34)

Orthodox social policy tends to approach questions of need from the perception that they should be gauged in practical terms with regard to satisfaction; that is, for example, an individual in unfit housing does not need adequate housing to the same extent as the person who has had their house burnt down (Spicker 1993: 12). However, the perspective being outlined here would suggest that despite the described situation, this does not mean that the individual in unfit housing does not need proper housing. Clearly, as Spicker notes, the need for proper housing remains in both cases, although we might argue that the person who has their house burnt down might have plentiful resources to find other accommodation (or another home), whereas the person in unfit housing may be relatively 'trapped' by their lack of resources. The overriding point is that the need for adequate shelter exists and we run the risk of getting sidetracked if our discussion of needs and rights is centred solely on which claim of need is worth more than another. The latter approach leads us away from universalism and towards the kind of mechanical relativism that imposes upon people the obligation to show why their perceived need should be satisfied rather than accepting that people should be empowered to look after their own needs to as great an extent as possible. The 'needs as claims' position relies heavily on the measurability of human need which, from the post-industrial socialist perspective, is difficult to gauge, especially when it comes to 'beyond survival' needs. The fact that existential needs are hard to measure does not negate their integrity nor the idea that individuals should be able to satisfy them. In asserting the primacy of the principle of autonomy Weale captures the thrust of this argument:

> [T]here is one overriding imperative to which government action ought to be subject in the field of social policy, and that is the principle that the government should secure the conditions of equal autonomy for all persons subject to its authority. This principle of autonomy asserts that all persons are entitled to respect as deliberative and purposive agents capable of formulating their own projects, and that as part of this respect there is a governmental obligation to bring into being or preserve the conditions in which this autonomy can be realised.
>
> (Weale 1983: 42)

This takes us into slightly different territory from orthodox social policy thinking as it suggests that rather than professionals mediating between the claims of different individuals (which may in any case be expressions of their wants), our guiding principle should be enabling individuals to take more control over their own need satisfaction. Self-determination for autonomous individuals and greater opportunities for people to engage in collective self-determination in social groups then become the key to general need satisfaction. Post notes that these ideas have been a traditional foundation in Leftist thinking on needs:

> [I]nequalities of power raise issues of needs which necessarily transcend existing social relations. Thus, we may postulate a need for autonomy, by which is meant the capacity to satisfy wants in conditions of equality and mutuality, without domination by an Other. Autonomy may therefore be seen as a need which fuses and transcends the others; like them it is socially expressed. Morality and rationality should . . . sustain the autonomy of the individual.
>
> (Post 1996: 64)

In this theory of needs, then, there is undoubtedly importance placed upon the satisfaction of survival needs such as shelter and food, but they are regarded ultimately as contributors in the process of developing individual autonomy. Moreover, the reciprocal obligations which are implied in this need-based conceptualisation of autonomy form the basis of Post's defence of an expression of basic needs as rights alongside other rights such as to experience mutuality and to live in a condition of order. Thus: 'If these are violated, then autonomy is denied and a condition of injustice exists' (Post 1996: 64). This would suggest that the pursuit of autonomy goes hand in hand with the quest for social justice – it is an ongoing process not an end-state goal. The Left-libertarian perspective is concerned with providing individuals with as much control as possible over their need satisfaction and hence their autonomy because 'unmet needs . . . impair agency' (Goodin 1988: 48–9). This would involve basic social rights which would contribute to the process of developing autonomy rather than essentially guaranteeing that needs for autonomy would be met. In Freeden's words: 'Total autonomy is as chimerical as total welfare; hence less than perfect autonomy must be regarded as a social and political inevitability' (Freeden 1991: 53). In this scenario our proposition for state welfare becomes one in which individual autonomy is maximised within the constraints that are placed on individual autonomy by the principle of social justice. This must curtail autonomy to some extent in redressing imbalances in opportunities to act autonomously. This reflects the Left-libertarian perspective in which the experience of autonomy is flawed when the social context in which one acts is not populated by other autonomous individuals. In this sense the need for autonomy is neither a claim against material resources, because it does not lend itself to tangible measurement, nor a direct foundation for the imposition of social rights, because the latter are actually indirect determinants of autonomous action. Welfare, if it is to be gauged by the standards of need satisfaction, must take into account 'beyond survival' needs rather than those associated with survival alone. In short, our perceptions of welfare need to stretch further than the effects and operation of the welfare state. The upshot of this theory is that 'rights fall short of, rather than exceed, the bounds of need' (Jones 1994: 154). In the words of Taylor:

> Citizenship rights and entitlements must be tied to a fulfilment
> of need. Need in this respect can be seen as dynamic and dif-
> ferentiated, as against the universal and abstract basis of rights.
> The meeting of need . . . implies not just a set of rights but the
> power to achieve needs, in terms of access to resources. Needs
> can only be satisfied in an active process of human develop-
> ment, both individually and socially. The concept of citizenship

tied to the idea of the right to satisfy need becomes dynamic, political and comes into a confrontation with power.

(Taylor 1996a: 163)

State welfare is linked to the satisfaction of survival needs as it is designed to provide minimal standards of living (however successful it is at doing so) for those who do not have the means or wherewithal for achieving those standards themselves as long as they fulfil whatever criteria define eligibility. In this sense we can currently equate survival needs with conditional social rights. The post-industrial Left argues that those needs should be met unconditionally given that the eligibility criteria of advanced capitalism are usually associated with work requirements of one kind or another. Identity needs such as autonomy, however, cannot be guaranteed by social rights and financial entitlements as traditionally understood because they are not always quantifiable and therefore 'any set of rights founded upon basic needs will be infected with similar indeterminacy' (Jones 1994: 153). Our only potential expression of rights and duties in relation to identity needs is that we have a right to self-determination as long as we are prepared to contribute to the self-determination of others. Put another way, post-industrial socialism believes that the fullest extension of autonomy is best guaranteed by a new politics of time in which individuals have the rights to a limited amount of work and the opportunity not to have to spend the majority of their time in activities which are linked to work. The obverse of this coin is the related duty to work for only a limited amount of time to allow the redistribution of working hours to others and also to be prepared to contribute one's labour to the furtherance of one's society.

This conceptualisation transcends the boundaries which are often erected in theoretical debates over needs such as 'thick' and 'thin' perspectives (Drover and Kerans 1993a: 11–13). Thin perspectives on needs are those which provide objective and universal theories that imply moral obligations to need satisfaction such as that of Doyal and Gough. Thick perspectives tend to promulgate the notion that we need to comprehend the varying contexts in which needs are experienced and satisfied. As such 'the "populist" sensibilities of the thick theory approach and the critique of positivism which underlies them are an important counter to welfare "knowingness"' (Soper 1993: 71). Where the former approach is universalist and, for Soper, verges on the precipice of prescriptive bureaucracy and welfare professionalism, the latter is more pluralistic and, in terms of need satisfaction, particularist in practice. Clearly, in the advocacy of identity needs such as autonomy, Left-libertarians such as Lodziak are promoting universal needs which correspond with 'thin' theories and pluralist need satisfaction which fits with the 'thick' approach. Thus, as Drover and Kerans (1993a: 11) suggest, these theories are 'interdependent and complementary rather than oppositional'. However, as Soper argues, we need to be sure that there are some governing criteria in which we gauge need satisfaction particularism (Soper 1993: 73) because it is fairly obvious that thick theories could result in a quagmire of relativism. In terms of post-industrial socialism the key foundational principle and governing criterion of measuring different forms of need satisfaction is self-limitation (Gorz 1993), which implies some guarantee of economic well-being to enable individuals to lead a less materialistic existence. Our position with regard to needs and rights is summed up neatly by Plant:

> [R]espect for persons requires us to respect not their particular view of the good but, rather, the capacity of a person to pursue such a good – namely, the capacity for agency . . . [T]his capacity requires resources as well as forbearance. We cannot both respect a person's moral capacity and be indifferent to whether he or she has the means on which the realization of that capacity depends. This means that respect requires that the person be provided not with the specific means to meet specific goals but, rather, with the basic goods of agency that are required for the pursuit of any good at all.
>
> (Plant 1988: 71)

Taking this perspective on board, we can summarise the position as it stands for developing options for a post-industrial socialist welfare theory. This involves six key points:

- Left-libertarians such as Marcuse and Lodziak argue that perceptions of need are socially constructed but also that the inability of advanced capitalist societies to meet needs engenders emancipatory potential.
- The social construction of needs does not negate the importance of the conceptualisation of human needs as has been the case with Doyal and Gough, especially when it comes to providing a foundation for debates over the levels of benefits.
- The fact that we can outline a universal theory of needs does not preclude the advocacy of particularistic means of need satisfaction for different social groups – this is a slightly more pluralistic perspective akin to that of radical democrats than Doyal and Gough's theory.
- Needs do not automatically translate into social rights, although this

may be the case with such survival needs as food and shelter – however, it is unlikely to extend to existential or 'beyond survival' needs such as the need for autonomy. Nevertheless, Jordan highlights the continued centrality of autonomy in arguing that 'roles and relationships in every sphere should start from a basis of equal *autonomy*' (Jordan 1987: 149).

- The level of social rights does not by necessity have to be sufficient to cover all human needs because it is impossible to put a price on the amount sufficient to guarantee autonomy – thus the levels of benefits are likely to vary between, for example, different countries and eras, which means that they will be decided through political and economic negotiation (Weale 1983: 36–7).

- In this sense rights contribute to the development of personal autonomy but genuine fulfilment necessitates the empowerment of individuals so that they can take as much control as possible over their own need satisfaction.

Ultimately, the post-industrial Left position argues that the development of personal autonomy entails a subversion of the ideology of work and a new politics of time which breaks the link between income and work. In short, this means nothing less than the end of work-based society. To analyse the implications of these goals it is essential to identify the utility of social and economic policies which are most relevant to post-industrial socialist theory. The most obvious theoretical models which fit the criteria outlined above are those which embody some form of guaranteed income, which we must turn to next.

5

BASIC INCOME

A viable theory for post-industrial socialism?

Despite the existence of ideas relating to basic income in the history of political thought, such as in Tom Paine's *Agrarian Justice* (Purdy 1988: 198; Robertson 1996; Vallentyne 1997: 328), it is generally regarded as a new dimension in modern political theory. Thus in recent years there has been a substantial growth in literature concerned with universal, unconditional welfare policies such as the basic (or citizen's) income and the integration of taxes and benefits (Van Parijs 1992c, 1995; Walter 1989; Parker 1989; Little 1997; Clinton *et al.* 1994). While much of this work has been developed by Left-libertarians, Greens and feminists (Offe 1992; Parker 1993; Pascall 1997), basic income theory also provides food for thought for liberals and even those of a more conservative bent, depending on which format it takes.

This chapter will attempt to establish the utility of basic income theory for post-industrial socialists and the potential effects that such a policy might bring about. In so doing we will see that basic income might be a partial solution to the problems in advanced capitalism which are identified by post-industrial socialists, but that wider radical policy initiatives (notably in economic policy) would also need to be put in place to fulfil the emancipatory objectives of post-industrial socialists.[1] Basic or citizen's income debates have been much more thorough in the rest of Europe than in the United Kingdom (Loftager 1996; Loftager and Madsen 1997; Andersen 1996; Milner and Mouriaux 1997) and there is growing currency for the idea among academics (Van Parijs 1992c) and groups such as the Basic Income European Network. The next step for advocates of basic income is to attempt to popularise radical policy proposals among groups such as trade unions which, given their productivist legacy, are not the natural constituency of post-industrial ideas (Gorz 1989a: 219–42; Little 1997; Coenen 1993). As David Purdy points out, basic income is a project which could engender partnership between a range of groups, including trade unions, in pursuit of more radical social and economic policies (Purdy 1988: 266).

Basic income is usually presented as a guaranteed income paid to each individual regardless of any past or present work requirement. As such it is usually presented as a beautifully and disarmingly simple idea (Van Parijs 1992a: 3). While this is ostensibly a reasonable comment, once the surface is scratched a more complex theoretical debate begins to emerge.[2] Many of the intricacies of basic income rest firmly upon the ideological approach which analysts bring to the debate with regard to the concepts of equality, liberty and social justice, and the consequent perspectives on the role of the state in social and economic policy. In turn this has a further effect on perceptions of community and citizenship which are employed by basic income theorists.

The variety of basic income theories will be examined in the coming sections which will be followed by an exposition of a post-industrial socialist critique. The chapter will conclude by suggesting that basic income theory provides a potentially radical solution to the problems evident in the new economy (Little 1997), but that there is little inherent reason why it necessarily should foster socialist outcomes. This is reinforced when critics of socialism such as John Gray claim that basic income may be part of 'a policy aiming to reconcile the human need for economic security with the destabilizing dynamism of market institutions' (Gray 1995: 113; see also Gray 1993). Alternatively, post-industrial socialists such as Gorz claim that basic income policies could only generate socialistic outcomes if they are accompanied by a planned reduction in working hours and a right to work (Bowring 1996: 113). Indeed, even neo-Keynesian, social democratic commentators such as Will Hutton have admitted that a redistribution of income may not be sufficient to resolve our economic and social problems; we might actually require a redistribution of work (Hutton 1996: 24).[3]

Exploring basic income theory: liberty and equality

Initially, it may be worthwhile to outline a working definition of basic income. Van Parijs suggests that it is a particular type of guaranteed minimum income but it also differs from the types of minimum income currently guaranteed in some European welfare states. This is because,

first, basic income is strictly individual, given to all people on an individual basis irrespective of their household situation; second, it is given to all irrespective of income from other sources (labour income or capital income); third, basic income is not subject to whether people are willing to work. It is not restricted to the involuntarily unemployed, but it would be paid to people who choose not to engage in paid work (for example, housewives, househusbands, students and tramps).

(Van Parijs 1997b: 5)

From this the attraction of basic income to a philosophy based on 'the end of work-based society' should be apparent. The ideas put forward by Van Parijs[4] could theoretically sit comfortably with an economy which cannot guarantee that sufficient jobs will be created to ensure that there are enough jobs for all. Clearly, a basic income guarantee could enable individuals to spend time away from the formal economy of work for wages in order to engage in self-ordained activities. In this sense it can be presented as an appropriate strategy to combat a situation in which Europe was beginning to experience 'a kind of mass unemployment which could not be interpreted as conjunctural or cyclical in nature but which rather resulted from central features of our socio-economic system' (Van Parijs 1997b: 9). Basic income theory also fits into a developing Left-libertarian perspective which rejects several defensive notions of full employment, such as the traditional Keynesian framework (and consequently the Keynesian welfare state), the relatively full employment promised by market liberals (so long as the level of employment is not deemed to be inflationary, however that is defined), or the perspective that the state should intervene to create more proper jobs (as understood within the dogma of the ideology of work). To this extent Offe *et al.* suggest that a 'return to the apparently "normal" model of a society of work and wage labor insulated by a welfare state is (a) economically undesirable, (b) ecologically indefensible, and (c) socially unacceptable' (Offe *et al.* 1996: 209).

A critique of Van Parijs

The basic income theory that Van Parijs defends rests heavily on the unfair distribution and appropriation of resources (especially accessibility of work) in advanced capitalist societies and the need to redistribute income to offset the unequal maintenance of those scarce resources such as labour. Thus his position suggests that 'where natural or other kinds of social resources are scarce, agents who appropriate them owe rent (a kind of tax) for the appropriation' (Vallentyne 1997: 327). Van Parijs presents a broadly (though not strictly) egalitarian proposal based upon a theory of justice which promotes individual self-ownership, real (that is, resourced) liberty and a requirement that 'the social pot be spent so as to *leximin* the values of the opportunities open to each member of society, that is, to maximize the value of the least valuable opportunity set' (Vallentyne 1997: 334–5). Put more simply, Van Parijs believes that all the things 'which we receive in very unequal amounts should be distributed in such a way that those who have the least of them should have as much as possible' (Van Parijs 1997b: 12).

In the era of mass unemployment the inequality of labour resources can justify the payment of a basic income to all which does not stigmatise or marginalise those who do not have access to work for wages (Van Parijs 1997b: 14–15). For this reason Van Parijs rejects the common criticism that basic income schemes provide a *carte blanche* for freeriders who want to take the basic income without contributing reciprocally to society. However, this idea translates suspiciously into the notion that it is defensible to deprive people of their chance to contribute to their society as long as we compensate them in a pecuniary fashion. Arguably a more satisfactory means of assuring a more equitable distribution of resources would be to redistribute work. This kind of allocation would require much more substantive economic policy initiatives than would the Van Parijs scheme and undoubtedly it would require a longer time scale for implementation and planning. Moreover, the ethics of a redistribution of work would require justification as it seems that it would mean less work for those currently in employment. None the less, this burdensome task is defensible for the post-industrial Left because unconditional basic income schemes such as that of Van Parijs seem to be founded on the principle that forced exclusion from work for wages can be justified as long as there is some kind of financial remuneration. Van Parijs is well aware of inequalities in labour resources and his solution is founded on a theory of justice which believes that a pecuniary settlement is needed to provide 'the basis of a fair distribution of these resources that will empower people: especially those at the bottom of the talent and human capital hierarchy' (Van Parijs 1997b: 15). The problem with this viewpoint is that it provides no challenge to the existence and reproduction of 'the talent and human capacity hierarchy' but merely compensates people when they are marginalised, excluded or unlucky enough to find themselves at the bottom of the hierarchy for whatever reason. A more thorough challenge to the hierarchy would be to guarantee individuals decent work regardless of their place in the hierarchy, to guarantee a mode of social insertion and social inclusion for all. However, this goes far beyond the liberal egalitarianism of Van Parijs.

Perhaps the key criticism to be made of Van Parijs's welfare theory is that it does not focus on aggregate social welfare but concentrates instead on transfers that will provide the greatest value for the worst off. Hence the theory of justice at work centres explicitly on the condition of the worst off. In the words of Vallentyne:

> It is crazy to hold that one should help one person moderately instead of helping many other needy people more. The problem with the leximin is that it gives absolute priority to the worst-off person(s). A more plausible view would agree that a worse-off person has some priority over a better-off person without claiming that this priority is absolute in the sense that any benefit (no matter how small) to a worse-off person has priority over any benefit (no matter how great) to a better-off person.
>
> (Vallentyne 1997: 341)

The value in Vallentyne's approach is that he appears to have a broader conception of the meaning of aggregate social welfare than Van Parijs, who relies too heavily on a legalistic understanding of the politics of egalitarianism.[5] That is, the former makes a clearer attempt to elucidate the complex interplay between self-ownership and equality whereas the latter presents a theory which remains within the formal realm of philosophical argument. A stronger commitment to social welfare – understood as an egalitarian philosophy which goes beyond mere monetary resources and the lack thereof experienced by the very worst off – must be formulated for a genuinely Left-libertarian approach. Van Parijs provides a formal theoretical defence of basic income without developing strong ideas on what provides a society or community with welfare. He doesn't centre enough on the types of resource which need to be redistributed to ensure social inclusion and security. From a post-industrial socialist perspective, it can be argued that the formalism of Van Parijs's liberal egalitarianism glosses over the mechanics of an integrated society. For example, while Van Parijs can defend the payment of sums of money to surfers who do not contribute to the production of social wealth (i.e. on the basis that they are not allowed to commandeer scarce resources to make profits) on liberal egalitarian grounds, this does not necessarily explain how opportunities are going to be created to allow surfers to get involved in the generation of social wealth if they so desire (Van Parijs 1991). In other words, formally enshrining a right to an income regardless of contribution can be liberatory and egalitarian to some extent but does not go far enough in terms of redistribution. Indeed, there is considerable scope for basic income to be appropriated by neo-liberals to reduce state responsibilities for social welfare. By running down the levels of basic income, the Right could maintain a façade of equality while simultaneously strengthening the relationship between welfare and paid work. The latter would be required by individuals receiving a low basic income to augment their income to satisfy needs. The post-industrial Left prefers to concentrate on the importance of redistributing work to promote social inclusion for all, which, as we shall see, has strong implications for our perception of liberty and equality.

The other key objection that is raised in relation to basic income theory is that of the freerider – the individual who receives an income generated by the fruits of the labour of others and does not contribute to the generation of social wealth (Van Parijs 1992a: 8 and 1997a; White 1997). This objection is rejected by Van Parijs on the grounds that individuals should actually be compensated for the appropriation of scarce resources by others rather than demonstrating their eligibility for paid work. White, on the other hand, raises the objection that 'payment of a substantial UBI [unconditional basic income] . . . will lead to the exploitation of productive, tax-paying citizens by those who, while capable of working, instead choose to live off their UBI' (White 1997: 312). White is not opposed in principle to the distribution of natural resources (subject to some criteria), but is more concerned with Van Parijs's claim that jobs are resources which also should be justly distributed and, therefore, that the absence of that distribution requires compensation in the form of basic income.

The post-industrial Left extracts something from both sides of this debate. André Gorz has argued that in social terms we do nothing for integration, stability and solidarity by excusing people from working on the grounds that others hold a disproportionate amount of the work available (Gorz 1992). This position accepts Van Parijs's argument that work is a resource which has a value such that it should be redistributed in the perfect world. However, Gorz goes further than Van Parijs in suggesting that it should *actually* be redistributed. At the same time the issue of reciprocity which is raised by White is also a feature of Gorz's approach. The latter argues that the performance of socially necessary work is a reciprocal obligation of citizenship which corresponds indirectly with a guaranteed minimum income. This is in line with White's proposal that a 'reasonable work requirement' should be introduced into basic income proposals (which would, in effect, negate their definition as an unconditional basic income).

> [T]he egalitarian conception of reciprocity implies that in return for this decent minimum of income each citizen has a corresponding obligation to perform a decent minimum of contributive activity, the size of this minimum varying with the

degree of productive handicap. We may refer to this as *baseline reciprocity*.

(White 1997: 319)

While this seems to be a reasonable position in defence of an egalitarian view of reciprocity, there is, given the constraints of the post-industrial economy, a problem in making guaranteed incomes directly correspondent with work performed (as that work is currently unevenly distributed) – a problem also evident in Baker's theory of compensating differentials (Baker 1992; Little 1997; see below). Moreover, from a liberal egalitarian perspective, it can be argued that individuals should have a choice over when they perform their work requirement, although this principle increases the possibility of freeriding occurring. However, the rationality of freeriding is assumed in the manner of rational choice theory that the utility maximiser would automatically choose not to contribute when, on the other hand, it is equally reasonable to argue that it is perfectly rational for people to want to participate and contribute to the collective good – that utility may also be derived from undertaking activities which aren't automatically obvious in the theoretical fog of *homo economicus* (Rothstein 1996: 99–106). As we shall see in the following chapter, the citizen's wage proposal favoured by Gorz attempts to circumvent the problems addressed by both Van Parijs and White by combining their positions in the interests of individual autonomy, collective self-determination and equality.

Liberals and egalitarians

A Left-libertarian approach to basic income must address the question of what extent of self-ownership and self-determination can be limited by the constraints imposed by egalitarian thinking, as there may be some necessary trade-off between liberty and equality (B. Barry 1992: 140). Most approaches to basic income, however, tend to see it as a means of achieving 'the equal distribution of the capacity to make effective choices which constitutes genuine freedom' (Norman 1992: 147; see also Norman 1987). In this sense the trade-off is much more limited than Barry's view, and, using the ideas of Cohen, we can begin to identify a position whereby we retain features of autonomy and equality and some sense of self-ownership without prioritising the *principle* of self-ownership (Cohen 1995: 119). In other words, a practical political position on these issues will suggest that a pure concretisation of equality, liberty, autonomy or self-ownership will never come to fruition and that the key to alternative political proposals must be the promulgation

of a better balance of these concepts than is currently the case. It is on
this foundation that basic income theorists can speculate on the complicated relationship between taxation and social justice. Hillel Steiner
suggests that in terms of income there are three just forms of taxation
which can be defended on an egalitarian basis, while still coming from a
libertarian perspective. The first 'just tax is a tax on nature' (Steiner
1992: 82). This correlates to some extent with Van Parijs's view that those
who do not appropriate scarce resources are rightfully compensated for
the use of those resources by others. Similarly, Steiner defends the right
to tax the historical appropriation of natural resources which were originally commonly owned. In the terms of the debate this seems a
reasonably uncontroversial point because 'non-users must be so compensated because the jointly owned resources are made less available to
the non-users, given the use made of the resources by the users.
Compensation is required to make up for the fact that the jointly owned
resources are at least partially used up when they are used' (Carling
1992: 94).The second just tax promulgated by Steiner is a tax on the
estates of deceased people which he justifies by comparing bequeaths
with gifts and arguing that bequeathers retain significant powers over
those who benefit from their benevolence as opposed to those donating
gifts. Moreover, there remain significant power differentials and legal
relational variables between bequeathers and their executors in terms of
rights and obligations (Steiner 1992: 84–5). Steiner deems that dead
individuals are, in a way, returning to nature and are therefore liable to
'a use-compensation tax' because their estate returns to an unowned
(natural) condition (Carling 1992: 94). The third just tax rests upon the
notion that the libertarian defence of our self-ownership must

> attribute some intelligibility to the idea of a person's labour,
> and regard various unagreed takings of them as unjust. The
> paradox arises from the simple fact that each of us, as a non-
> primordial moral agent, is the product of other moral agents'
> labour . . . [H]ow is universal self-ownership even possible?
>
> (Steiner 1992: 86–7)

In other words, how can we present individuals as self-owning moral
agents when our moral agency is closely tied to the historical development and labour of other moral agents? Does this not suggest some
degree of interdependence, at least with those whose toil produced the
goods (or attributes) that we now claim as our own? The extent of this
principle is debatable, as Steiner uses it to suggest that his third just tax
would be 'a tax on children's genetic information. Parents of children

114

with more valuable genes are liable to pay a higher tax' (Steiner 1992: 88). In other words, Steiner regards the activities and attributes that children acquire from their parents as 'natural' resources which can be dealt with in a similar manner to the position apropos nature which provides the foundational basis of his other two taxes. Thus it seems that parents are to be taxed as if their genetic information was a 'pure public good' (Carling 1992: 95), that this information was totally unaffected by the use of others. Carling rightly suggests that genetic information is not something that is given up on the point at which individuals attain self-ownership (whenever that is deemed to be) and therefore is not a sound entity to be justly taxed. None the less, he does suggest that the appeal to egalitarianism should provide a fruitful location from which to resource basic income proposals to accompany the appeal to basic income on libertarian grounds.

None the less there is considerable disagreement between egalitarians on the utility and effects of basic income theory which are linked to the different conceptions of equality that are at work, such as equality of opportunity, outcome or treatment (Norman 1992: 148–50).[6] The complexity of the problem of equality with regard to basic income is highlighted by Baker, who defends 'the moral force of equality of outcome' but also highlights the vast difference between equality of outcome and a basic (equal) income when it comes to the different needs and burdens that individuals may bear (Baker 1992: 105–7). He clearly envisages basic income being set at a level that is sufficient to cover basic needs (along with other basic income advocates such as Bill Jordan). Given that need satisfaction (though not necessarily broad genetic categories of human needs) will vary from individual to individual, Baker proclaims that an egalitarian basic income would also need to vary likewise.[7] In other words, an egalitarian basic income would have to fluctuate between different individuals in order to provide greater equality of outcome. Thus Baker proposes a theory of 'compensating differentials':

> If everyone worked the same hours at identical jobs, equal income might arguably continue to represent an equal outcome. But if people do different kinds and amounts of work, constituting different kinds and degrees of burden, equal income will no longer suffice. Equality is restored only if the burdens of work can somehow be balanced off against the benefits of income. That is what a system of compensating differentials tries to do.
>
> (Baker 1992: 108)

The strength of Baker's approach for the post-industrial Left lies in his emphasis on work as well as income. Rather than just viewing welfare as a financial entity, he suggests that we also need to acknowledge that work has a particular burden and effect on individual welfare (and, we might add, social welfare in general). From this perspective we are well advised to evaluate activity in the economic sphere as especially influential on our well-being in collaboration with whatever financial transfers are arranged by the state. In effect what Baker proposes is a scheme whereby the onerous and negative burden of work is compensated by a financial payment (which is deemed to be good and beneficial). Thus the more onerous and burdensome the work an individual performs, the more recompense is due to them in terms of basic income. Given the differences between individual burdens, this, Baker believes, is the only means to ensure equality of outcome. This may be true but this formulation is highly problematic for the post-industrial Left because it strengthens rather than weakens the links between income and work. Indeed, in a way, Baker's basic income is *defined* by the work that is performed, which makes it unsatisfactory in Left-libertarian terms, although he provides ample economic evidence of its appeal in terms of equality of outcome (Baker 1992: 111–15; Little 1997: 49). Having said that, Baker does provide a solution to Van Parijs's problem of freeriders and basic income. Where Van Parijs is content to justify the right to a basic income in terms of use and compensation – 'compensatory justice' (B. Barry 1992: 130), Baker's compensating differentials theory avoids freeriding altogether because 'equal burdens are equally rewarded, while unequal burdens are compensated for by unequal benefits' (Baker 1992: 122). Thus two conceptions of basic income related to equality emerge: the formal egalitarianism of Van Parijs based on unconditionality and a liberal approach; and Baker's compensating differentials which reflect egalitarian concerns with equal outcomes. Neither perspective concurs with the desire of the post-industrial Left for 'the end of work-based society' because the former is explicitly unconcerned with inequalities in labour markets, preferring monetary compensation over the redistribution of work, and the latter is too concerned with evaluating actual work and providing compensation which would formally strengthen the relationship between income and work. There is a strong temptation to reach the conclusion that 'a system of basic income would create a society that was markedly unequal because of the gap that would have to be created between those on the basic income and those in employment' (B. Barry 1992: 140).

Basic income, community and society

A different dimension to basic income theory is provided by the burgeoning debate on communitarianism as exemplified in the ideas of some radical democrats such as Bill Jordan (1987, 1989, 1992, 1994, 1996). In a large body of work spanning twenty-five years Jordan has been the most vociferous advocate of basic income in the United Kingdom, despite the fact that this debate has been much less prominent there than in other European countries. Most importantly, where much basic income theory is located within the confines of political philosophy and economic theory, Jordan provides a much needed sociological defence with regards to issues of poverty and social exclusion.[8] Despite his respect for the philosophical rigour of Van Parijs's contribution to basic income theory, Jordan argues that his advocacy of basic income rests too heavily on formal, liberal rights which are divorced from untidy realities of social welfare linked, for example, to work situation, domestic household arrangements or other social inequalities (Jordan 1994).[9] Jordan suggests that, while the ethical justification of basic income through the abstract usage of liberal notions of the rational individual may be necessary, a sociological justification of basic income must involve analysis of patterns of labour distribution and the effects of the lack of paid work for many on social life in general. In this scenario basic income is promoted as part of a broader package which is designed to reinvigorate communal life, make decision-making more accountable and participatory, and, generally, to inspire a 'radical, egalitarian communitarian' reappraisal of democracy.

Nevertheless, Jordan appears to place great faith in basic income as a key catalyst in his radical egalitarian communitarianism and a central policy strategy in the promotion of 'the common good' as a rejuvenated focus for radical politics (Jordan 1989). Accompanied by a fairer distribution of public goods, basic income is envisaged as a means through which communities and groups can become collectively self-determining and the individuals therein can become more autonomous. This involves an overt attack on social exclusion and the marginalisation of the 'underclass' which, Jordan argues, has no common interests with those in the economic sphere (Jordan 1989).[10]

> The case for basic income as a response to the underclass phenomenon rests . . . on two features. By ameliorating (eventually eliminating) the poverty trap, it would give the excluded minority access to the market system of fairness by reward for effort, and hence to savings, property and other private goods. But

also, by giving everyone a universal share of resources on the grounds of membership (citizenship), it would be a mechanism for including all in the common good.

(Jordan 1992: 172).

What Jordan means by a 'mechanism' is not immediately clear – certainly basic income could involve some notion of the common good but, simultaneously, in the liberal guise, it could merely formalise individual rights which, as Jordan acknowledges, can exist independently with no regard to commonality and co-operation. Indeed, as Gorz notes, one cannot guarantee full membership of society and community or the common good through a pure financial transaction of redistribution (Little 1997). From this perspective, Jordan's earlier (1992) strategy appeared to involve a leap of faith in which social inclusion and cohesion can be generated or at least accentuated by a pecuniary solution: that is, the basic income guarantee.

However, more recently Jordan has modified his position in reaction to Van Parijs's abstract liberal theory. Like post-industrialist socialists such as Gorz, Jordan has recently suggested that individuals should be in a 'process of renegotiating the fairer distribution of burdens and benefits, work and leisure, which Basic Income would make possible' (Jordan 1994: 121). While Jordan has always advocated these ideas within his general framework, he has never previously tied them in explicitly with his perspective on basic income. He does not want to make basic income conditional on the redistribution of work but argues that this redistribution needs to take place anyway, presumably for the common good. In this scenario basic income is more of a limited enterprise in financial redistribution than a proactive social policy designed to bring about the common good rather than merely encourage it. This seems moderate in the overall scheme of things (clearly Jordan is not presenting basic income as the panacea for all our ills) but one is left wondering where the impetus for actually engineering the appropriate conditions for the common good to flourish are going to come from.

While it seems appropriate within the framework developed here to support Jordan's proposition that individuals should have duties to 'work' in their communities, there still appears to be a leap of faith as there is little indication as to policy proposals which would enforce this rather abstract 'duty' which Jordan envisages. If basic income is not a fundamental part of how we understand these duties, then their political manifestation looks problematic. As Lister notes, 'he does not really explain how one moves from his economic analysis to the political changes required' (Lister 1997: 90–1). While Lister's point is valid in

this case, the comment is a fairly standard objection to basic income proposals. Of course, manifold political and economic proposals have been
suggested regarding the implementation of basic income policies (Parker
1989). Rather, as Offe notes, the main point for proponents of basic
income is to formulate a strategy in which an alliance can develop built
around a broad package of social, economic and political ideas which
include basic income (Offe 1992: 74; 1996: ch. 10; Lodziak 1995).
Undoubtedly, despite the reservations outlined above, Jordan's work is of
central importance to the furtherance of that strategy.

Towards a non-productivist alternative on welfare

For Offe, an alliance must be built around Left-libertarian philosophical
ideas and the variety of perspectives which have sought to challenge the
capacity of welfare capitalism to guarantee universal citizenship. In this
sense he proposes a coalition of groups which seek to formulate radical
theories, and economic and social policies which can provide an alternative welfare settlement – one that is non-productivist and, therefore,
opposed to the ideology of work. This, he argues, must be the fundamental basis of a new social policy consensus. While such a consensus
may be difficult to achieve politically, Offe provides salient reasons why a
basic income could not only decouple income from work in a positive
manner but also rejuvenate the way we work in welfare capitalist societies.

> It does not seem too far-fetched to assume that in wealthy indus-
> trial societies, employees who are accorded the right to
> withdraw from paid work without penalty and at the cost only of
> loss of income (but not poverty!) will as a result be better moti-
> vated, better qualified, and in a better physical and psychic
> condition to engage in it (for then they would be choosing it
> 'voluntarily') than those from whom this choice is withheld,
> and who must consequently work knowing that nonengagement
> in paid work (or the failure of an attempted engagement in it)
> carries the threat of material need and social stigma.
>
> (Offe et al 1996: 219)

This thesis hinges on the differentiation employed by Offe to exemplify
the hegemony of productivism and his desired non-productivist alternative. Here it is worth returning briefly to the productivist assumptions
(mentioned in Chapter 2) which he argues encapsulated a syndrome of
the 1970s and 1980s which can now be brought into question in welfare
debates (Offe 1992: 68–9). Offe rejects the family basis of welfare

capitalism in which households are viewed as the primary sources of welfare and the units by which eligibility for welfare is the major concern. A second theme following from this assumption which Offe also criticises is the notion that each of these family units would contain a breadwinner providing sufficient funds for the family which would minimise the extent of claims on state welfare provision. Moreover, he notes the breakdown of corporatist systems for establishing collective decisions and the capacity of the welfare state to meet all the residual needs which weren't met by family units or collective actors. For Offe, the disintegration of these productivist assumptions is the substance of the decline in the relatively consensual existence of welfare capitalism in the post-war years. Thus the amalgamation of these processes of delegitimisation has made these features of welfare capitalism increasingly distant and inapplicable to modern economic realities (Offe 1992: 69).

The decline of the assumptions of the productivist welfare state leads Offe to suggest that rather than resorting to the anti-collectivist 'catallaxy' of economic liberals, the selectivity of conservatives or the outmoded productivism of social democracy, the future path for welfare theory may lie in Left-libertarian ideas and basic income proposals.[11] On this understanding basic income is justified on the grounds that it is explicitly centred on a theory of citizenship which recognises the value of activity performed both within and outside the paid labour market. As such Offe envisages the key feature of basic income to be the fact that it would be a social policy which would be paid to all citizens rather than to (current, potential or previous) workers. Moreover, like Jordan and Baker but unlike Van Parijs, Offe suggests that the 'coverage of *basic needs* is the criterion of justice [for basic income]' (Offe 1992: 70) along with the sustenance that is provided by individual autonomy and collective self-determination.

Communities and the state: obligations and reciprocity

The problems of tying new welfare proposals to basic human needs have been addressed in the previous chapter, and will also be revisited in the next chapter but at this juncture it seems pertinent to indicate the impact of linking basic income to human needs with the relationships between the state, communities and individual citizens. On this point the theorists mentioned above have differing perspectives but it seems that Offe (1996) is much the most thorough. Although Jordan (1985) has previously written extensively on the role of the state, his more recent work has centred on communities as facilitators of the duties of citizenship which are implicitly linked to his more developed notion of basic income

(Jordan 1994: 121). Of course virtually all advocates of basic income retain a prominent role for the state (although this isn't necessarily the case with liberal formalists or economic liberal defenders of negative income tax) [12] but there has been little specific literature on the position of the state in terms of individual rights and obligations except to say that it will pay for basic income proposals. Rather, the role of the state tends to be evaluated in terms of the fiscal arrangements for funding basic income as opposed to outlining a proactive position for the state in which it plays a key part in engineering an inclusive society. This latter perspective is admittedly unpopular but it seems fairly clear that the post-industrial economy applies pressures to labour markets which act against the foundational principles of the productivist welfare state. If this is the case then a strong role for the state in providing aspects of social welfare seems inevitable.

Why, then, do commentators such as Jordan focus on communities as locations of welfare provision? The answer seems to lie in the fact that Jordan was among the most vociferous critics of the Keynesian welfare state in the 1970s and 1980s and the idea of the state as the locus of welfare provision remains a dangerous and potentially centralising solution. Nevertheless, while the defence of communities as sites of inclusion and fulfilment for individuals seems perfectly apt for basic income proposals (on the grounds that separating income from work opens up opportunities to spend time in communal or co-operative activities), the creation of the conditions in which communities are given a key role in the new welfare settlement must be guaranteed and facilitated by an entity with the jurisdiction to ensure that communities and localities are providing their welfare function adequately. This does not in itself lead us towards the *dirigiste* state (although it could) if it is envisaged as a state with powers considerably devolved to localities and communities. It seems the extent of this devolution is part of a pluralistic process of political negotiation in which communities, parties and movements such as trade unions must challenge the role of the state as a rather unsatisfactory provider of social welfare. Failing that, social welfare faces the prospect of a divided system whereby most citizens are faced with minimal provision in the state sector, which is constantly threatened by the vicissitudes of competitive markets, or expensive private schemes that are accessible only to those with an abundance of financial resources who can buy out of state provision. In terms of relationships between individuals, a system whereby welfare is recognised as a social value which we are all expected to participate in, providing for each other in a range of different types of community (which seems commensurate with the values of basic income theory), is more favourable than the privatisation of welfare which leads to welfare being understood as something individuals pay for (and insure against) in formal contractual relationships with private companies. In other words, the role of the state in guaranteeing social welfare need not lead to *dirigisme* or Keynesian-style interventionism in the economy – the issue is whether the state is capable of dispersing power appropriately.[13] As Taylor-Gooby reminds us:

> A government which seeks to expand autonomy thus has to be active in the limitation of inequalities of power, and operate to minimise the impact of social values which sustain them . . . [T]he form of state provision may differ. It may include a pluralism of method. However, the obligation on government to guarantee needs-based rights continues, and this may lead to the extension rather than the curtailment of the scope of state intervention in social life.
>
> (Taylor-Gooby 1994: 85–6)

The propensity for empowering communities is evident in Jordan's basic income theory (though not necessarily in Van Parijs's conception), not least because it is envisaged as a means of enabling people to participate in democratic life. In the words of Healy and Reynolds: 'As the individual needs the resources to sustain physical life, so too resources are needed so that she/he can participate in the life of the community' (Healy and Reynolds 1995: 53). However, there are key debates and issues that emanate from this over whether basic income can *ensure* participation, or more radically, whether basic income should be *conditional* on participation. On the former point this seems highly unlikely. It is highly optimistic to suggest that giving people a sum of money will automatically ensure that individuals get involved in local decision-making or communal life (Little 1997). Indeed, as Gorz has suggested, a basic income scheme could become a subsidy for low-paying employers and drive down wages because employers could benefit from using casual labour as people sought only to top up their basic income. Certainly, basic income theories are not designed to undermine the position of the weakest in the labour market further but it is quite possible that this would be the outcome. As such, basic income theories by themselves do little to challenge the dualisation of the labour market and the growing splits emerging between core and peripheral workers. In this situation there is absolutely no guarantee that basic income would ensure healthy communities and active citizens.

The second issue of conditionality and participation is more philosophically pressing. Jordan correctly challenges Mead's 'new puritanism' which promotes 'workfare' in the USA (Mead 1985)[14] on the grounds that there is little theoretical credence in the idea that there must be direct correspondence between the rights we are granted and the duties we owe, although this does not mean that we don't owe duties at all (Jordan 1994: 107–8).[15] Moreover, Jordan critically compares Mead's perspective with that of Locke insofar as property and self-ownership appear to be the key to Mead's view of obligations of citizenship: 'those with property incomes have no obligation to work for the community . . . [but] claimants of state support owe it to taxpayers to do work in return . . . [T]hose who claim the community's assistance forfeit some of the civil rights enjoyed by "independent" citizens' (Jordan 1994: 119).

As we will see, a model of obligatory participation is a central aspect of post-industrial socialist theory and one that Jordan has come round to. However, in impressing that rights and duties need not be directly reciprocal (which is broadly correct) he loses focus over how obligations are to be undertaken, and any concrete notion of reciprocity. Jordan rejects the views of Gorz and Opielka which indicate that our obligations are reciprocal in nature with the rights we receive: that is, they are inherently related to the state. For Jordan, obligations of citizenship 'should be set in the actual communities – the kinship networks, groups, unions, movements and neighbourhoods – in which people belong' (Jordan 1994: 121). Gorz accepts that much more activity needs to be undertaken within communities in the micro-social sphere that Jordan outlines above, but also that individuals should participate and work in a wider sphere, a larger community, to ensure social insertion. After all, in practical terms, our rights are not ordained by communities but by the state or larger international bodies. This being the case it seems reasonable to locate our (indirectly) reciprocal obligations on this macro-social level as well. For Gorz, this obligation should take the form of the performance of socially necessary work. Of course, as Gorz reminds us, not all jobs are economically rational and in many cases the work that is performed in the public sphere is not efficient in the sense that it might be cheaper if some jobs and excessive working hours were reduced and redistributed (Gorz 1989a,1994). Jordan also makes the highly pertinent observation – similar to Offe's anti-productivism – that participation in labour markets is not necessarily an efficient or desirable phenomenon in itself. On the contrary, it may well be extremely inefficient, especially as technological developments could lead to a decrease in the amount of labour necessary.

The conclusion of this discussion of basic income and community suggests that communitarians need to be clearer about the role of the state in welfare provision. The changes required by a basic income policy cannot be imposed without a co-ordinating role for the state (in conjunction with communities and institutions of civil society) and certainly communities cannot manage basic income by themselves. This provides a challenge for orthodox communitarianism because, as Goodin notes,

> the welfare state is neither necessary nor sufficient nor empirically particularly crucial to the realization of the communitarian ideal. Communitarian values do not justify the welfare state uniquely; they may not justify the welfare state at all . . . [T]he sort of generalized altruism that communitarians seek may be an impossible dream built on an untenable analogy to village society.
>
> (Goodin 1988: 118)

Of course, this does not mean that the post-industrial Left should ignore appeals to community but that the concept should be analysed in a more thorough manner, especially with regard to the relationship with the state and society as a whole. These issues will form the basis of the discussion of a participation wage or a citizen's wage in the following chapter.

The political economy of basic income

One of the most desirable features of the majority of basic income proposals is that they would simplify the massive and complex bureaucratic arrangements that surrounded the Keynesian welfare state and the lack of clarity which is engendered by the failure to integrate (to whatever extent) tax and benefits coupled with the inability of the system genuinely to identify personal and social welfare.[16] To this extent Purdy argues that

> the idea is to consolidate all existing direct cash transfers payable under social security programmes – whether tied to individual insurance contributions or non-contributory, whether universal or selective; all indirect financial benefits in the form of various personal tax allowances; and all other state grants to persons such as student maintenance allowances and self-employment or small business subsidies.
>
> (Purdy 1988: 194)

There is a variety of reasons why basic income makes economic sense, from the eradication of means testing and targeting (with the massive accompanying bureaucracy) to the possibility that there might be a new definition of full employment which is more suited to the new, flexible (post-industrial) economy. The pressures on welfare states are particularly stringent in the 1990s with, in the United Kingdom for example, a squeeze on social security benefits which relies optimistically on the future creation of managed job growth to reduce the public expenditure bill through welfare-to-work initiatives (Little 1997) and a cash crisis in the health service amid unwieldy bureaucracy and a new managerial culture (Jordan 1994: 121–2; Clarke and Newman 1997). The amount of recent research into the feasibility of basic income schemes has been pursued more vigorously by radical economists than political philosophers and sociologists, not least because if a blueprint for state welfare was needed and a blank page was provided, few would come up with the various models of the welfare state that are currently in place throughout the world. This problem is explained eloquently by Robertson:

> In industrialised countries awareness has been growing that our existing systems of taxes and welfare benefits are perverse – economically inefficient, socially unjust and divisive, and ecologically damaging. Taxes on income, employment, profits and added value penalise the contributions which people and organisations make to society. They tax people on the value they add, not on the value they subtract. By raising the costs of employment, they increase the levels of unemployment, thereby causing waste of human resources and many social problems.
>
> (Robertson 1996: 550)

In this climate there is an opening whereby the political economy of the welfare state can be reassessed. To this end three main issues need to be addressed by the post-industrial Left. First, it must ask whether a basic income accompanied by a new tax regime would be more efficient than current welfare arrangements. Second, it must assess the feasibility of integrating taxes and benefits. Finally, it needs to clarify methods of funding basic income schemes in order to assert their viability.

Rethinking efficiency

The issue of efficiency is complicated insofar as the degree of efficiency of any welfare regime remains open to interpretation as long as there is little agreement about the role which state welfare and taxation is supposed to play (Creedy 1996). For example, different perspectives on efficiency in the United Kingdom welfare state emerge from neo-liberal thinkers, who advocate the most minimal of safety nets, and contemporary reports such as that of the Commission on Social Justice outlining a future for the welfare state (Commission on Social Justice 1994; Little 1997). From the former perspective the welfare state can be viewed as a monolithic edifice which is inherently inefficient due to the provision of services for the undeserving poor, scroungers, single mothers, and so on, while the latter social democratic viewpoint holds that the welfare state does act as a useful remedy to the inequalities generated by contemporary labour markets but needs some modifications to preserve efficiency in the conditions that prevail at the end of the twentieth century. Basic income is questioned from both of these standpoints because, instead of centring welfare provision and services on those who are most in need, it suggests that maximal efficiency is generated by providing an adequate income guarantee for all. It is clear from most costings that the majority of basic income schemes would be more expensive than the welfare state as we know it now (although large sums would be saved from the abolition of existing benefits and bureaucratic welfare institutions). Given the attacks on the welfare state from a range of perspectives, it seems odd that basic income theories are defended on the grounds of efficiency when it seems likely that they would entail an increase in public expenditure and taxation. The key to understanding the basic income theory of efficiency is to recognise that what is efficient is deemed to be not what is the cheapest option but rather what is *the lowest cost option which is actually effective*. In this sense efficient social policies are not just those that minimise welfare spending but those that enhance social integration in a capable fashion. Moreover, such an understanding of social welfare may well reduce public expenditure in other areas.

Building upon these ideas, we can begin to outline a theory of efficiency which can justify basic income. The central feature of this theory is that individuals are empowered to take some control over their individual welfare, and in order to facilitate this growth in self-determination the state must provide a basic income guarantee which is not predicated on a range of conditions and qualifiers. This is what Goodin calls 'a minimally presumptuous social welfare policy' (Goodin 1992b: 195). The nub of this theory lies in the rather pragmatic contention that, although basic income can be defended on libertarian or egalitarian grounds, it can also be promoted on the basis that:

> Schemes that pay everyone an unconditional basic income are also less presumptuous than more conditional programmes of income support. They are *less presumptuous* not merely in the sense just canvassed – less prying and intrusive, and in consequence less

demeaning and debasing. They are less presumptuous in the
sense that they make fewer presumptions: they assume less about
the people whom they are aiding. And that makes basic income
schemes more efficient in one important sense than more conditional schemes of income support.

(Goodin 1992b: 195)

There are numerous ways of expressing this point but it is vital to note
that Goodin sets up his argument in terms of the very inefficiency of the
methods currently used in the targeting and means testing of benefits in
welfare capitalism and that this is what makes the welfare state presumptuous. In other words, the criteria for testing benefit eligibility are
'surrogates' which may be more or less adequate in providing efficient
social policies; Goodin concurs with Offe in noting that the changing
shape of work and domestic family arrangements have enormous implications for social policies which are means tested. The fact that social and
economic conditions are in a state of constant flux is deemed to be a
sound reason for developing less presumptuous social policies which do
not set conditions based upon work requirements or assumed familial
relationships. For Goodin, the need to reformulate state welfare provision should not be based upon specific sociological assumptions
(although these may be highly relevant in justifying basic income proposals) because 'sociological facts are uncertain, highly variable and, in
any case, constantly changing' (Goodin 1992b: 198). While Goodin is
aware of socio-economic developments, he prefers not to bring them
into his basic income equation, which is a valid but slightly perilous position as it could lead to the decoupling of basic income theory and
provision from the very developments which substantiate the claims of
advocates who must build a new coalition of support for it (Offe 1992).

An economic case for basic income?

The discussion of the role of the state in providing basic income as part
of a broader strategy of social and economic policies also establishes the
strong role that basic income could play in the wholesale reconstruction
of social and economic activities. An example of where socio-economic
conditions could be heavily influenced by a basic income is provided by
Standing, who notes that the decoupling of income from work would
provide an incentive for activities carried out in the black economy to be
brought into the public sphere, which, of course, would make them tax-
able. This is important in terms of the economic justification for basic
income because 'in so far as a basic income scheme encouraged "black

127

economy" work to become legitimate, the tax base would be expanded, so reducing the real cost of such a programme' (Standing 1992: 58). This is a point of some debate, as Clinton *et al.* (1994: 36) have argued that 'the high tax rates on earned income and acceptance of non-paid work status might increase the incidence of "informal economy" working.' While there is some currency in this point, the post-industrial economy is, as Standing notes, not reliant on mass employment, and the minimisation of paid work could be deemed desirable. However, this has a fundamental knock-on effect on tax revenues to be collected on incomes – a problem that poses key questions for basic income theorists but which post-industrial socialists such as Gorz and advocates of a participation income such as Atkinson (1995) might avoid. None the less, it is important to recognise the advantageous socio-economic implications of guaranteed income schemes to provide a broad picture of why they are gaining new advocates (and to counteract the standard and often ill-informed knee-jerk reaction that they cannot be afforded).

Standing points to other socio-economic benefits of basic income proposals such as the decline of the 'poverty trap', although it must be said that it would not be eradicated and that in some conceptions high marginal taxes would ensue. However, he correctly notes that basic income is far from a recipe for mass inactivity and indolence because people work for a variety of reasons and not just the income accrued from work (Standing 1992; see also Dore 1996). Other advantages that Standing identifies include greater labour flexibility, more self-employment, less institutionalised stigmatising unemployment and greater opportunities for those that are deemed 'retired' on a rather arbitrary basis. Moreover, it would open up opportunities for greater sexual equality in work, not just with regard to work for wages but in the domestic sphere. In other words, basic income may be a strategy for decoupling income from work, but a vital by-product of any thorough debate on basic income is the re-evaluation of the activities we perform and the rethinking of our work–leisure combinations. Thus Standing comments that

> a citizenship income scheme could facilitate labour flexibility through providing income security. If so, it would surely be preferable to the supply-side approach of flexibility through lower wages and selective means-tested benefits for the lower paid – a combination that automatically destroys an incentive to work.
>
> (Standing 1992: 59)

Nevertheless, it is essential to identify potential economic problems that might arise with regard to basic income, given the advantages outlined by Standing and Goodin above. The major point that needs to be assessed initially is whether the integration of taxes and benefits which is part of basic income theories is a workable option for social and economic policies. To this end Clinton *et al.* (1994: 32–3) provide a useful analysis of basic income in their contribution to the Commission on Social Justice. Their model encompasses the following features of a basic income proposal:

- it would involve full integration except for housing benefit and disability;
- it would be paid on an individual basis;[17]
- the period over which income and tax would be assessed would be the current year;
- there would be a uniform rate (although see note 17);
- all citizens would be entitled to basic income (although a definition of citizenship may be problematic);
- one agency would oversee basic income and taxes (although there would be a separate body for housing and disability benefits);
- it would be financed by abolishing many existing benefits, tax breaks and reliefs along with the elimination of expensive administration and higher taxes.

Clinton *et al.* quickly point to obstacles to a *full* basic income such as cost and the removal of work requirements before noting that, despite probable costs, the implementation and administration of basic income would be 'reasonably straightforward' given the organisations that already exist (this is not necessarily the case with a partial basic income).[18] Moreover, they note a range of social advantages that derive from basic income proposals, from the prevention of poverty (depending on what level basic income would be set) through redistribution and individual independence to income security throughout. The authors do, however, record potential political problems with basic income, such as the potential loss of up to 80,000 jobs in the United Kingdom civil service as the tax and benefit systems were simplified. For the post-industrial Left, though, while this might cause economic problems in terms of funding basic income from income tax revenue, politically it is less problematic as, of course, post-industrial socialists view the decline in bureaucracy and the redistribution of working hours as potentially emancipatory developments. In the words of Clarke and Kavanagh:

A Basic Income scheme is the first step in the move towards a post industrial definition of work and labour. As jobs become

more like assets than inputs, it will become increasingly important to develop mechanisms in which they can be more
efficiently and fairly distributed. This will entail a change in the
notion that a full-time job is a forty hour a week paid job.

(Clarke and Kavanagh 1995: 114)

Conclusion: basic income and post-industrial socialism

Before going on to outline conceptions of participation income schemes
or the citizen's wage it is important to take stock of the post-industrial
socialist perspective on basic income theory. In brief, the position is one
whereby the development of the post-industrial economy makes basic
income a viable option. Indeed, the provision of a basic income guarantee could actually be a key facilitator of mature post-industrialism in the
sense that the problems associated with the decline of meaningful, paid
labour would be minimised by a substantive state-backed financial settlement. Moreover, basic income seems appropriate in the context of the
sociological changes that have come about in advanced welfare capitalism
which are far removed from the conditions in which the original post-war
welfare settlement was formulated. To this extent some Left-libertarian
commentators such as Offe and Jordan have come out in favour of basic
income, as have liberal egalitarians such as Van Parijs. Importantly, each
of these commentators expresses an interest in basic income as part of a
process towards a different kind of social organisation – in other words,
basic income isn't presented as an end in itself but rather as a step
towards the development of a different type of society. These ideas have
been substantiated by the work of economists like Parker, Purdy and
Atkinson who, in demonstrating the feasibility and relevance of radical
ideas on guaranteed minimum incomes, have shown that basic income is
no longer on the periphery of welfare debates due to its perceived
expense. What, then, are the problems with basic income theory which
lead post-industrial socialists such as Gorz to object to basic income as an
essential strategy for the future of welfare? There are five main reasons
why the post-industrial Left might question the utility of basic income:

• While basic income clearly could protect individuals from the harsh
  outcomes that are generated by the flexibility of the new economy, it
  might also reinforce the effects of the new economy by institution-
  alising the marginalisation of large groups of people from the secure
  elite at the apex of the economy.

130

- Ostensibly, basic income supports individuals who can't find work, but equally it could subsidise employers who want to exploit workers with low pay – safe in the knowledge that each individual had a basic income to back up their wages.
- Thus basic income theories can be criticised for using social policies to solve the problems generated by the new economy without actually getting to the nub of the problem which is the inability of governments to formulate economic policies which would provide ample security, equality and liberty for those in the merry-go-round of flexible labour markets.
- Basic income advocates may suggest that the decoupling of income from work performed is likely to result in a growth of activity in the voluntary community sphere but do not identify clearly enough how community relations are going to be developed sufficiently. In other words, the pecuniary measures associated with basic income cannot, by themselves, regenerate the concept of community and a more forthright and clearly defined role for the state is necessary.
- Basic income clearly does not provide equality of outcome but does provide some concessions to egalitarianism while retaining a strong libertarian dimension. However, it would provide little equality with regard to the distribution of work and guarantees limited liberty for individuals when it comes to the work they want to perform – in other words, it might enable individuals to exist without work but it does not provide any firm promises of paid work for those who don't have a job but who want to contribute their labour to the generation of social wealth.

All of these quibbles with the effects of basic income theory do not equate to a wholesale rejection of guaranteed income proposals. Indeed, while the ideas which will be outlined in the next chapter will be shown to be more attuned to post-industrial socialist ideas, it is unlikely that these proposals could be put in practice without an interim period in which a basic income guarantee was in place. Nevertheless, it also clear that post-industrial socialists envisage a different and more radical type of guaranteed income scheme than a solitary basic income (Little 1997). Gorz gives three main reasons why this is the case. First, work must be reduced for everyone with the decline in earnings being compensated by a social income. Second, the redistribution of work which would be facilitated by a reduction in working hours would have to be accompanied by a range of educational and training programmes to allow the unemployed and marginalised to take up the newly created jobs. Finally, any proposal to promote activity in the voluntary or community sphere must also be supported with the growth of and developments of facilities – spatial, technical, and so on – to enable communities to flourish. Thus basic income schemes are useful to the development of post-industrial socialism if they are part of an integrated range of social and economic policies. André Gorz provides the backdrop for the next stage of the argument when he states the case for a post-industrial socialist approach:

> [A]ccess to work in the public sphere is essential to economic citizenship and to full participation in society. In complex modern societies, the participation in the social process of production is an essential factor of socialization and of membership in socially formalized communities and groups, even if working time is reduced to less than half the present average.
>
> (Gorz 1992: 182)

6

THE CITIZEN'S WAGE AND REDUCED WORKING HOURS

In the last section of this book the focus will move on to the alternative welfare proposals which correspond most clearly with the Left-libertarian philosophy that underpins post-industrial socialist thinking. The exposition of the post-industrial Left perspective so far has identified why more orthodox approaches to the welfare state are problematic in the context of the new economy. Attempts have been made to articulate new socialist approaches to some of the recent developments in the economy, such as the promotion of market socialism, for example, or the advocacy of the potential of post-Fordism, but they have been shown to be just as problematic in outlining an avenue beyond the current impasse as are theories such as orthodox post-industrialism and post-modernism. The evaluation of the traditional critiques of the welfare state and theories of citizenship in order to highlight the validity (or lack thereof) of traditional ideas have shown their relevance in the development of a coherent post-industrial socialist position on the future of welfare. Thus, having identified the utility of a blend of ideas developed from the traditional critiques, it has been possible to outline the potential of a cogent theory of human needs from which a reinvigorated state welfare programme could be devised. From this basis the most dynamic and sophisticated proposal which fits the 'post-industrial' features of the new economy – that is, the demise of traditional conceptions of work patterns – has been the variety of conceptions of a guaranteed basic income which attempts to break the work/income nexus. However, at the end of the last chapter it was argued that basic income was a viable notion in terms of a break between income and work but that there was little evidence that this fragmentation would be clear enough.[1] In this sense it was suggested that basic income might fit with a limited notion associated with the post-industrial economy but that the development of a genuinely post-industrial socialist society might require more thoroughgoing and radical ideas.

This chapter will examine some of the alternative strategies for welfare put forward both by elements of the post-industrial Left such as Gorz (1994) and others such as Atkinson (1995) who share the aspiration to reform the welfare state but suggest different policy proposals. There are three main questions for post-industrial socialists which arise from the problems with welfare capitalism and the suggested alternatives to it that have been outlined already:

- What might the features of post-industrial socialist social policy look like given the critique of more traditional approaches?
- What would be the relationship between these social policies and economic policy?
- What principles would be embodied within these new policy networks?

To address these questions, we will begin with an examination of André Gorz's advocacy of a citizen's wage, which will be compared with both basic income proposals and notions of a participation income. This will involve an analysis of notions of participation and conditionality and their place within post-industrial socialist ideas. Then the focus will broaden to examine the importance of a socialised economy in which the state presides over an economy which has the reduction of working hours as a central dynamic. Finally, these ideas and policies will be evaluated with regard to Left-libertarian concerns with liberty, equality, solidarity and social justice. Thus the aim of the following analysis of post-industrial socialist ideas on welfare is to set out a framework through which Left-libertarian philosophy can be concretised into coherent policy proposals. In the words of Rainer Land:

> [S]ocialism is a society which evolves in such a way as to create growing spaces for the development of individuals in the fields of material civilization, work, the environment and consumption ... A style of life and consumption which is rich but makes small demands on natural resources, which allows a great many varied subcultures to develop and expands the scope for individual autonomy – these are the emerging values of a new conception of rationality. It will become a reality when all economic decision-makers develop their strategies and determine their decisions on the basis of the felt needs and lived interests of individuals themselves in their democratic organizations, associations and initiatives.
>
> (Land, cited in Gorz 1994: 41)

André Gorz and the citizen's wage

Gorz has come to be seen as one of the most influential Leftist political thinkers in Europe in recent years (Little 1996). Moreover, his thorough analysis of economic developments, his investigations into the politics of work and welfare, and his heretical approach to the sacred cows of socialism have marked him out as the archetypal post-industrial socialist theorist. Having been one of the first Leftist commentators to engage with political ecology in the 1970s, it is not surprising that Gorz was one of the first advocates of a guaranteed income (albeit not an unconditional, basic income scheme).[2] The difference between Gorz's proposals and those of most advocates of basic income is that the former argues that a genuinely liberatory guaranteed minimum income must be accompanied by a reduction in working hours for all so that opportunities can be expanded to provide work for everyone who wants to work at any given time. Thus Gorz (like most basic income advocates) wants to break the work/income nexus, but he is also adamant that this fracture should not entail a work/individual break which would increase the ruptures which are evident in contemporary flexible labour markets. In other words, a guaranteed minimum income is to be retained but not at the expense of those who are already existing on the periphery of the domain of employment. From this perspective it is both libertarian and equitable to provide individuals with an income regardless of their current work performance, but it is not socially just to use the existence of this income as an excuse for maintaining inequitable labour markets with all their harmful effects on social inclusion and integration.

Gorz's stance is augmented by a very specific conception of citizenship. It is based on the notion that full citizenship entails the opportunity to contribute to the maintenance of communities and society as a whole, and to participate in the generation of social wealth. This, he argues, requires individuals to have a blend of different activities including work in the domestic sphere, in communities and in the wider public sphere. This latter activity is most likely to take the form of work-for-wages whereby individuals acquire an identity and social insertion from the work they perform. For Gorz, autonomous individuals must be given choice over exactly when and where they perform this work as it must be recognised that many activities have intrinsic value in themselves without necessarily having to be rewarded in the form of remuneration. This kind of thinking is what Lodziak (1995) refers to as a 'new politics of time' – the notion that individuals should have greater self-determination over the blend of activities they perform and that collectively there should also be power to debate the organisation of the state, communities and civil society democratically. From this perspective some of the problems of basic or citizen's income should be evident. No such reorganisation of the politics of time is inherently attached to basic income proposals and, in practice, they would be wide open to abuse from low-paying employers, neo-liberal governments and those who benefit from the dualisation of the labour market, that is, elites in secure full-time employment who owe their positions to our institutionalised acceptance of sharp divisions between core and peripheral workers. Thus it would seem that proponents of a citizen's income such as Purdy are misguided in recommending it as a means of reviving social citizenship precisely because it would be unconditional (Purdy 1994: 33). Post-industrial socialists such as Gorz contend that it is only by making conditional social and economic policies that we can properly direct them towards appropriate ends. With regard to a citizen's income, conditions would have to be placed on the state and employers (to provide sufficient employment opportunities for those who want to work at a given time) and individuals (to perform an amount of socially necessary work in a given period) in return for a 'second cheque' from the state which would recognise an individual's contribution to social goods.

Conditionality and participation

From an economics perspective, Atkinson also suggests that some form of conditional participation (although not necessarily in the paid labour market) would be necessary to justify an 'active citizen's income' or participation income because 'it will be difficult to secure political support for a citizen's income while it remains unconditional on labour market or other activity' (Atkinson 1996: 67). The issue of popular support is central to this debate because, as Purdy notes, neo-liberal ideas have become almost hegemonic in the pursuit of not the most efficient welfare settlement but the cheapest one – no matter how inefficient – that we can get away with before social disintegration and disorder ensues. These ideas suggest that we are close to a boundary beyond which serious problems will develop unless we begin to formulate comprehensive welfare reform. In this scenario Purdy is on a sound footing in arguing that there is 'no need for BI [basic income] supporters to be apologetic about "high" taxation ... [although] they will have a hard time persuading their fellow citizens that the price is worth paying' (Purdy 1994: 41). At the same time it is worthwhile repeating that advocates of basic income need to be forthright about the savings that would follow on from the eradication of means testing and bureaucracy, and the notion that a less presumptuous welfare settlement might well be more efficient.

From this it seems clear that there are several shared aspirations between supporters of an unconditional basic income scheme and those who advocate a degree of conditionality. Both concur that there are inherent problems with the welfare state in advanced capitalism in practice and in philosophical terms. This is most clearly manifest in the profusion of means testing and targeting in order to reduce the bill for public expenditure. Atkinson (1996) notes that the downside of widespread means testing includes the growth of poverty and savings traps which often derive not just from individual circumstances but those of the family in which we live; the fact that take-up rates of stigmatising means tested benefits are poor, which clearly must be manifest in the efficiency of the welfare state to solve the problems that justify its continued existence; and the way that family-gauged benefits mitigate against our institutionalisation of independence and individual welfare. Thus he suggests that 'means testing is economically inefficient, provides an incomplete safety net, and takes social policy backwards rather than forwards' (Atkinson 1996: 68). These criticisms echo the arguments developed by Goodin in attempting to formulate a new minimally presumptuous route for state welfare which does not misuse resources in the name of more 'efficient' targeting (Goodin 1992b).

Taking these perspectives on board we can begin to clarify the conceptual framework in which Gorz develops his notion of a citizen's wage. His position is clearly more presumptuous than that of Goodin insofar as Gorz identifies that individuals need to contribute (in the broadest sense) to their communities and society at large to be eligible for the citizen's wage. However, this is not envisaged as a workfare arrangement whereby benefits are directly paid on condition of performing (often unpleasant) work. Rather, it assumes that individuals will want to contribute to the development of the society they are part of without necessarily working full time as we know it. In this sense individuals are also to be rewarded for working less because, in working fewer hours, we are opening up opportunities for other people to work as well. In other words, by reducing our working hours we can help to include those who are currently excluded and marginalised from society. As we shall see below, Gorz believes that higher rates of productivity could offset some of the loss of individual income which would be a by-product of reduced working hours and simultaneously provide the revenue to finance a citizen's wage which would help to maintain income levels that would have decreased due to working fewer hours (Gorz 1994: 102–17). To put it another way, the citizen's wage would be a payment made by the state to each individual who undertakes to perform some socially necessary work but not so much as to limit the opportunities for others to contribute to society – it is just as much conditional on not working as it is on working, and in that sense it is remote from notions of workfare. Within democratically arranged parameters it is up to the individual to decide which blend of time she or he finds most appropriate at any given point. For example, parents may want to spend more time with their children at certain times and should be allowed to do so in the knowledge that that time is not regarded as less important than time spent in work-for-wages but is, in fact, seen as socially useful. Likewise, individuals should be able to contribute to collectively determined projects in their communities and in civil society without suffering from a lack of an adequate income. Clearly, then, Gorz's ideas are not designed merely to promote a more pragmatic welfare state in which work is redistributed or to enable people to avoid participation and contribution, but rather they are motivated by a desire to promote individual autonomy, collective self-determination and an emancipatory politics of time.

> [T]his time may be used however one likes, depending on one's situation in life, to experiment with other lifestyles or a second life outside work. In any case, it limits the sphere of economic rationality. It has a socialist significance in so far as it is combined with a social project that puts economic goals in the service of the individual and social autonomy.
>
> (Gorz 1994: 76)

Evidently Gorz's proposals contain an element of conditionality which separate them from wholly unconditional basic income schemes. However, it should be equally clear that this conditionality is tied into a Left-libertarian philosophy which promotes the idea that individuals should contribute to society (in a range of different ways). Thus the citizen's wage can be viewed as more emancipatory and liberal than basic income schemes because the latter would do little to challenge the institutionalised divisions of capitalist labour markets and would openly compensate individuals for their exclusion – indeed, Gorz sees a guaranteed income as a reward for 'compulsory passivity' (Gorz 1985: 40) – whereas the former encompasses a right to work and a right not to work at a given time which would facilitate individuals with proper choices over the organisation of their time. This would give individuals greater opportunities to find the most suitable blend of their time between work-for-wages, unpaid work (including that in the domestic realm) and leisure. This negates the myth that conditionality is inherently illiberal and the idea that conditionality must involve means testing or direct work requirements. Because a citizen's wage encourages participation more than basic income, it can be seen to be more genuinely emancipatory insofar as it would provide individuals with more autonomous choices and ensure access to a limited amount of paid work over the course of a lifetime.[3] The downside of this argument is that it might need more planning and bureaucracy than the simple organisation of a wholly unconditional basic income but at the same time it would undoubtedly be less bureaucratic than the current means testing welfare state. As we know, bureaucracy contributes much to the cost of any welfare system and this aspect would make the organisation of the citizen's wage more expensive than basic income. At the same time, however, because the citizen's wage would guarantee access to some paid work when it was required, we might envisage that it could be set at a lower level than basic income which could offset the cost of bureaucracy.

The other issue related to the citizen's wage which may unsettle proponents of unconditional basic income schemes is the notion of participation, which could be viewed as a means of excluding people from eligibility for the minimum income. Post-industrial socialists would concur that direct criteria of eligibility (e.g. a specific work requirement at a given time) are likely to marginalise those who find it difficult to find work in the contemporary climate. Nevertheless, it must be noted that, in terms of the immediate political agenda (in the United Kingdom at least), ideas such as Atkinson's participation income have been more influential than unconditional basic income (Commission on Social Justice 1994: 261–5). One of the reasons which Atkinson gives for proposing a participation income is purely pragmatic: that political support is more likely to be generated by a conditional system (Atkinson 1996: 68). This may be so but it does little to challenge the neo-liberal hegemonic position whereby individuals have to prove eligibility for individual benefits rather than the onus being on the state to provide social welfare. Thus, while understanding the concrete political reasons behind this dimension of Atkinson's economic proposal, it does little to further our philosophical perceptions of the actual reasons for having welfare at all and, as such, does not in itself justify the principle of conditionality. He is on a surer footing in suggesting that participation is a desirable feature, especially in conceptualising the policy in relation to a notion of 'active citizenship'. This would allow a participation income to be paid to those who want to contribute part-time work but are unlikely to in the current regime because they would lose benefits. Atkinson also incorporates those who are unemployed but available for work as participating, which is more problematic from a Left-libertarian approach, as we shall see below. Thus Atkinson suggests that:

> The condition involves neither *payment* nor *work*; it is a wider
> definition of social contribution . . . The determination of these
> conditions would be different from those involved with income
> support at present: for example, an unemployed person who
> undertook part-time work would be qualifying rather than the
> reverse.
>
> (Atkinson 1996: 69)

This is a vital principle which differs from both the system as it stands and unconditional basic incomes. The former penalises individuals who want to participate (especially in unpaid work) and the latter compensates the unlucky while ostensibly reinforcing divisions in the labour market. None the less, Atkinson's proposals also pay insufficient attention to the inequalities which are ruthlessly doled out by flexible labour markets. For instance, the existence of a participation income could drive down wages as employers (especially those that provide low pay anyway) realised that workers gained a supplement on top of their wages to boost their income, although the extent of this trend might vary depending on the level of a minimum wage. Also the notion that it would be paid to those who were unemployed but available for work could provide a recipe for the continued marginalisation of the long-term unemployed – a neo-liberal government might well use the existence of a low-level participation income as a basis for keeping the long-term unemployed in their place, thereby leaving the economy to operate relatively unencumbered by high public expenditure on unemployment. Moreover Atkinson's approach seems less liberal than Gorz's ideas because the former would not provide opportunities for individuals to spend time without participating while still receiving an income, and it would not guarantee individuals the opportunity to participate and contribute to society. As mentioned above, it could actually do the opposite in the wrong hands. Thus Gorz argues that the

> guarantee of an income independent of a job will only bring
> freedom if it is accompanied by the right to work for everyone;
> that is, the right to participate in the production of society, in
> the creation of socially desirable wealth, the right to co-operate
> with others in the pursuit of our own goals.
>
> (Gorz 1985: 40)

One last point which Atkinson acknowledges is the idea that a participation income might actually change the economic behaviour of people in the sense that they might alter their actions to ensure their eligibility (Atkinson 1996: 69). This clearly could be the case and there is little doubt that many in the political sphere would be aghast at the thought of people leaving jobs in the knowledge that a participation income would be paid to them as long as they were merely available for work. Nevertheless, Atkinson is correct to affirm that even that scenario would be more effective than the profusion of means tested benefits which underpin social security in the United Kingdom at the moment. At the same time we might add that there is considerable evidence that people do want to contribute on a variety of levels in a range of different ways. As Dore suggests, 'the importance for self-respect of having a job . . . far outweighs its intrinsic importance in warding off boredom' (Dore 1996: 61). The point, then, for the post-industrial Left is to outline policies which would provide opportunities for self-respect which not only encompass paid work but also recognise the value in self-respect that individuals obtain from activities that are non-economic in a direct sense, such as being a good parent or developing artistic skills. Of course, these latter activities can be viewed as being economic in the sense that good parenting and teaching may result in the development of individuals who can contribute to the economy in the future[4] but, from a Left-libertarian perspective, it is appropriate to attribute values to these activities in themselves (in terms which have nothing to do with the economy but recognise that many activities are worthwhile whether they produce exchange value or not). In other words, there is value in terms of self-respect of 'having a job well done' even if it is unpaid and also of developing a skill in one's leisure time which one does not intend to put to economic ends, for example, in acquiring sporting skills without intending to become a professional, in learning a martial art without intending to use it for economic ends. This returns us to a notion of citizenship in which individuals achieve a blend of activities which are motivated by a range of factors from income to sheer enjoyment. What is clear is that economic rationality is not to be the central principle which guides human activity.[5] For post-industrial socialists, the sphere of economically rational activities needs to be severely limited, which entails a large reduction in working hours.

Reduced working hours and the socialised economy

André Gorz has been a long-time advocate of reduced working hours, although his motives have been much misunderstood (Little 1996; Bowring 1996). He does not believe that all work for wages is unpleasant and, contrary to the ideas some of his more vibrant critics, he actually

POST-INDUSTRIAL SOCIALISM

argues that it is in the interests of everyone to work for wages in the public sphere. This, according to Gorz, is the main means for individuals to acquire a sense of social identity and social insertion in modern societies (Gorz 1992). This is not to say that work-for-wages should be the primary activity in human life or that, even where there is not enough work to go around according to the dominant distribution pattern, it should still govern the life of everyone whether they are fortunate enough to work for wages or not (as is the case with the proliferation of the ideology of work). Rather, Gorz views work-for-wages as one type of activity among many. It may have different ends, principles and values from other activities but it is not in itself superior. It gives people identity and belonging in society but it cannot guarantee space for individuals to undertake autonomous activities, nor does it ensure that individuals are able to develop relationships with others in communities or associations of mutual interest. None the less, with amounts of meaningful, economically rational work in decline due to technological developments, advanced capitalist societies still revolve around work-for-wages to the detriment of other spheres of activity. Post-industrial socialists see the reduction of the amount of hours any individual can commandeer for themselves as a potential pathway for egalitarianism as it is only through the redistribution of work that everyone can be guaranteed the opportunity to partake in socially necessary and economically rational work. Thus Gorz's support for reduced working hours is not because he disapproves of work-for-wages. On the contrary he is much in favour of work in the public sphere and for that reason he believes that the redistribution of this work is the key for his brand of socialism.

From this perspective, access to the economy is not something that people who have work should take for granted. Like Van Parijs (1995), Gorz views work as a resource which is taken away from many and distributed inequitably. Where the former argues that individuals who don't have access to work should be compensated through a basic income, the latter argues that we need to intervene actively in the operation of labour markets to ensure that everyone has a full opportunity to undertake work in the public sphere if they so desire, as long as they do not work excessive hours. However, Gorz must also face the issue that some individuals (however few) may not want to contribute to the betterment of society and undertake activities in the public sphere. For this reason his approach appears less liberal than that of Van Parijs, which would entail some provision for 'freeriders'. Where the former would seem to have greater moral weight in terms of firm conditions for citizenship, the latter, it could be argued, is more genuinely universalist. None the less, it is the redistribution of work thesis in post-industrial theory which differentiates a formal liberal egalitarian approach (such as that of Van Parijs) and the emancipatory economic planning of the socialist egalitarian approach, and it also identifies the differences between the latter and attempts to resurrect neo-Keynesian economic management.

> Reducing working hours will not have a liberating effect, and will not change society, if it merely serves to redistribute work and reduce unemployment. The reduction of working hours is not merely a means of managing the system, it is also an end in itself in so far as it reduces the systemic constraints and alienations which participation in the social process of production imposes on individuals and in so far as, on the other hand, it expands the space for self-determined activities, both individual and collective. This development of free activities which are no longer work (in the sense this term has come to assume) obviously cannot be produced simply by reducing working hours. It requires a politics of time which embraces the reshaping of the urban and natural environment, cultural politics, education and training, and reshapes the social services and public amenities in such a way as to create more scope for self-managed activities, mutual aid, voluntary co-operation and production for one's own use.
>
> (Gorz 1994: 61)

This sets out a theory of reduced working hours which is clearly divorced from the new discourse of flexibility that dominates economic policy debates in the United Kingdom and the USA (Reich 1997) and the renewed calls for full employment (Smith 1997; Philpott 1997). Gorz's post-industrial socialism embraces notions of flexibility if it is to be enshrined in a way which empowers individuals to choose when they perform work in the public sphere. Such a view differs from dominant notions of flexibility whereby employers can hire and fire insecure workers on short-term contracts and governments use the demand for flexibility as a means to massage unemployment figures. Similarly, post-industrial socialists do not give up on notions of full employment – they merely reject the version of full employment which is propagated in the dominant ideology. However, full employment need not entail the idea that everyone is working for wages at any given time, an unlikely scenario in the contemporary era. Rather, one can argue that a policy of reducing working hours would allow work to be distributed more equitably and would be all the more effective if it was implemented within a climate whereby unpaid work and other autonomous activities were accorded equal primacy and value with paid work. In other words the ideology of full-time work as the apex of social activity needs to be superseded by a philosophy which recognises that much worthwhile activity takes place outside formal labour markets (Gorz 1994: 56).

Conceptualising the reduction of working hours

It is necessary, none the less, to identify what a policy of reduced working time might look like and what effects it would have. Purdy (1988: 151) identifies six forms which such a reduction could take:

1   a fall in standard working hours;
2   a fall in overtime;
3   longer holidays;
4   lowering ages of retirement or raising the age at which people enter paid work;
5   extended schemes of sabbatical leave;
6   a growth in job sharing with equity of rights for full-time and part-time workers.

Purdy recognises that these potential strategies for reducing working time find varying favour among employers and trade unions. For example, job-sharing and sabbatical schemes have not been as high on the agenda for unions and employers as some of the other options. This has been especially notable in trade unions in the United Kingdom but their counterparts in the rest of Europe have been much more involved in these debates, which could point to a source of regeneration for the movement here. The issues of overtime, the duration of holidays and early retirement tend to be the areas around which unions and employers have most dialogue over reduced working time. However, none of these measures *in itself* entails a move towards post-industrialism because all are inherently bound up with the existence of work-for-wages as the central determinant of social activity. This is not the case with a fall in standard working hours, though, if that reduction is channelled towards a new politics of time in which working time is planned through a socialised economy to ensure that work is more equitably distributed and that greater opportunities to contribute outside the domain of work-for-wages are created. Here we have another key to our definition of the principles of post-industrial socialism – *it is not just about reduced working time, it is about reduced standard working hours*. The reason for this is that the benefits of a reduction in working time alone can be subsumed within the economy by reducing the number of jobs rather than distributing the reduction within society by limiting the hours anyone can work, which should help the process of redistributing work.

> [I]ndustrialization has saved working time for everyone, throughout society, and the working time saved has been re-employed to a large extent *within* the economy to produce extra wealth which only industrialization enables us to conceive and create.
>
> (Gorz 1994: 48)

Thus, for Gorz, a reduction in working time will be relatively worthless in broader social organisation unless this decline in time spent working for wages is used to allow more people to contribute to the creation of social wealth. It is fairly clear that this socialisation of the process of reducing working hours could only take place within the context of socio-economic plans formulated and agreed by coalitions of governments, employers, unions and local communities. Gorz has sought to demonstrate how, under specifically planned introduction, a reduction in working hours need not reduce incomes substantially, especially if we are prepared to tolerate a low and steady rate of economic growth.[6] Moreover, we also need to adopt an *ex ante* approach to the process of reduced working hours which would provide us with a fresh opportunity for change, which is impossible if we take a traditional economic *ex post* perspective on designing political processes (Bowring 1996: 122). In other words, Gorz provides us with a programme of political possibilities rather than economic constraints on emancipatory progress: 'the point is to steer a process which is actually in progress by choosing the needs it is to serve. Either politics is the sum of such choices, or it is nothing' (Gorz 1994: 104).

What, then, are the choices which derive from the economic developments that Gorz believes are 'actually in progress'? He identifies four main proposals which he extrapolates from the rates of output and productivity in France in the early 1990s and the existence of a standard thirty-nine-hour week. Nevertheless, this type of calculation should be possible in the light of contemporary economic developments in any work-based country. Gorz identifies choices which could be made over a four-year period in which production is raised by 8 per cent and productivity by 12 per cent:

1 maintaining current working hours;
2 maintaining employment at current levels;
3 maintaining wages at current levels;
4 reducing working hours while increasing wages and the workforce.

(Gorz 1994: 105)

Under Option 1, which Gorz equates with current economic developments, the workforce will fall by 4 per cent because productivity is higher and the wages of those in work are likely to rise by about 12 per cent over four years. Under Option 2 wages would rise by 8 per cent while working hours could be reduced by 4 per cent due to increased productivity. Under Option 3 the increase in production by 8 per cent could theoretically enable an increase in the workforce by 8 per cent and working hours could be reduced by 12 per cent as more workers are employed and productivity is also increased. Option 4, however, is Gorz's preferred option as it is the only one which would encompass reduced working hours, the redistribution of working hours to those who are currently disenfranchised, and, crucially, *an increase in wages to offset the reduction in income which would ensue from fewer hours worked.* This latter aspect is vital for Gorz because he wants to develop a proposal which is attractive for all and this is part of the reason that he holds on to limited economic growth against Green arguments for zero or negative growth. While Gorz advocates limited economic growth to ensure his three-pronged economic proposal (fewer hours, a growing workforce, increased wages) and also to ensure some ecological restructuring at least for an initial four-year plan, he does not rule out more extensive ecological restructuring once the process and principles of reduced working hours are in place and the next plan is being developed. This outline of choices exemplifies the options that are available if we adopt an *ex ante* approach to socio-economic redevelopment and are prepared to enter into detailed multilateral dialogue over the formulation of a sustainable economic plan for a socialised economy.

Clearly, this kind of proposal is faced with considerable problems when it comes to implementation, not least because of the prominence of neoliberal perspectives on interference in labour markets in the United Kingdom and the USA. Potentially more fruitful ground can be seen in social policy circles in the European Union and in countries such as Germany and the Netherlands where the role of the state in guiding the economy is less controversial. However, one of the greatest problems for the post-industrial Left, if not the greatest problem, is in persuading the traditional agents of Leftist ideas such as the trade unions or socialist parties to take up the crusade for a planned, socialised economy (Coenen 1993; Little 1997). The unions, for example, in defending their sectional interests, are closely tied in with the ideology of work which permeates their relationships with employers. At the same time, the unions no longer tend to represent the people who would be the main benefactors of reduced working hours: that is, those who are currently marginalised from work in the public sphere. Having said that, the strength of Gorz's

146

position (Option 4), as opposed to the other choices he outlined with regard to the new economy, is the growth in wages to offset reduced working hours. It is this facet that he perceives as a key method of persuading the middle classes that they, as well as those who are currently disenfranchised, would benefit – a feature that Offe regards as essential to the process of popularising non-productivist social policies (Offe 1992). A proper discussion on the political choices which arise from the new economy would provide a space for debates on reduced working hours and the citizen's wage in which their broader advantages for all could be discussed. It is not impossible that individuals and organisations could develop a coalition of support for a proposal which had its roots in reversing the trends of marginalisation and exclusion that ensue from the 'flexibility' of the new economy. Indeed, support from a wide range of sources could be achieved for a vision of society which aimed 'not to produce the greatest possible wealth but to enable everyone to engage in productive and disinterested activities which ensure their place in society and their personal development' (G. Roustang, cited in Gorz 1994: 108). Moreover, reduced working hours would challenge the ideology of work and the proliferation of 'servant work' which characterises the development of advanced capitalism in the 1990s (Elliot 1997). In Gorz's words:

> A policy of RWH [Reduced Working Hours] implies that paid work is performed in the main by skilled persons who are well-paid, productive in the economic sense, and socially useful; it therefore implies that servant work, the aim of which is simply to do for others what they could just as well have done just as well in the same time, does not expand.
>
> (Gorz 1994: 110)

This section should exemplify the importance of reduced working hours to post-industrial socialist theory and it seems that Gorz has put it, rather than the citizen's wage, at the forefront of his proposals in more recent times. He refers to reduced working hours as the initial goal from which a citizen's income may develop in time. This seems reasonable in the sense that a radical social policy such as the citizen's wage would be extremely difficult to implement in an immediate fashion. On the contrary, an incremental implementation of the citizen's wage through a partial and then a full basic income scheme accompanied by reduced working hours may be the best way forwards. Nevertheless, Gorz has veered away from explicit mention of a citizen's income in his recent work – perhaps due to the misrepresentation of his work as a defence of basic income theory by a range of commentators (Bowring 1996: 112).[7]

The problem with Gorz's latter approach is that in neglecting social policy instruments for reversing the trends in the new economy, he leaves himself open to charges of economic determinism. This does a disservice to the broader perspective he has developed in most of his work, which recognises a twin-track approach to political change in which social and economic policy complement each other. Certainly, the post-industrial socialist perspective needs to promote issues related to economic democracy and economic welfare, but it also needs to be more forthright than Gorz in his most recent work about the most appropriate pathway for social policies.

Rethinking welfare and post-industrial socialism

In *Capitalism, Socialism, Ecology* Gorz refers to a possible policy of a 'second cheque' which he proposes as a compensatory payment to individuals who lose working hours and cannot have their wages supplemented by income from higher productivity. Clearly, this implies that the 'second cheque' would not be a permanent universal payment but one which individuals claimed when they were not working (or not working enough) to gain a sufficient income from work. While this may be compatible with a post-industrial socialism which guarantees an income to those who are not working due to their previous and/or future contribution to the creation of social wealth, it does seem to weaken the universalism which is clearly a strength of full basic income schemes. A break with this universalist ethos on social policy spells danger as it opens up opportunities for governments to engage in selectivist social policies which as we know from the experience of welfare capitalism can be highly ineffective and potentially stigmatising for those who receive welfare benefits. Undoubtedly, Gorz's moderated perspective is more immediately realisable in terms of policy implementation than a full basic income and he is correct to argue that 'the second cheque corresponding to the price of work which no longer needs to be performed will initially be the most attractive formula' (Gorz 1994: 112) when it comes to formulating social policy but, in the longer term, a universalist post-industrial socialist policy would need to reduce working hours more widely and thus *a full citizen's wage for all* would need to be developed in later economic plans, rather than just for those who cannot generate significant productivity gains. Moreover, increased production (even at the very limited rates that Gorz envisages) are likely to become more ecologically problematic as the years go by and in this sense higher productivity and output may become increasingly irrational. In this scenario a programme for post-industrial economic planning may move from an initial reduction in working hours, accompanied by a partial basic income which would increase as working hours were further reduced in the subsequent plans. Once working hours were reduced to a level whereby there were opportunities for everyone to work, then the likelihood is that a universal citizen's wage would be necessary to complement wages earned and to offset the fact that at any given time a significant number of people may not be engaged in work-for-wages. While Gorz is not explicit about this process, he has shown, most importantly, that in terms of economics, a citizen's wage policy is economically viable.

Welfare, the economy and social justice

In practical terms, of course, as with most economic theories, this kind of model could not be enacted exactly, as forecasting is notoriously difficult (as government budgeting would seem to prove). None the less, this does not invalidate the need for planning, as without it the operation of the economy would become anarchic. In other words, the fact that the operation of economies is difficult to predict does not mean that they should be left to their own devices, it means that efforts to regulate their operation should be all the more stringent. This is why even governments which promoted neo-liberal economic philosophies in theory, such as the United Kingdom and the USA in the 1980s, were never actually able to retract state intervention in practice. In this situation ideas such as the citizen's wage, basic income or reduced working hours become political decisions which governments will address in the future along with other economic choices. To quote Gorz:

> It is practically impossible . . . to forecast the rise in productivity with total accuracy, and select a corresponding RWH [Reduced Working Hours]. But the impossibility of doing this is far from negative in its implications: it demonstrates that the economy and the society cannot be managed on purely technocratic lines, and the choice of an RWH will always *initially* be a political decision. It is this which must be regarded as an independent variable. It is up to the economy to adapt itself to this, just as it adapted to the Sunday rest day, the eight-hour day, the forty-hour week, paid holidays, and so forth.
>
> (Gorz 1994: 112)

This suggests that the economy is ultimately subject to political control and must be organised and guided by political goals. In other words, the economy does not and cannot operate without political direction and it is up to decision-makers to decide the principles upon which that direction will be founded. In the current climate even governments which might be inclined towards potentially radical social policies remain imprisoned by homage to flexible labour markets and liberal interpretations of how the economy should operate (Marquand 1997). This is problematic as it is based on the conception that social policies and political decisions can only be formulated within the context of preordained liberalised markets, rather than creating social and economic policies in unison and recognising the fact that governments have some capacity to influence the operation of the economy (Leonard 1997). Thus politics is not just the domain of organising society, it is also the sphere of directing markets and regulating the economic system which is complemented by a range of other non-economic, but equally important, phenomena in civil society. The point for the post-industrial Left (and for those who might view this perspective as unrealistic) is that the economy does not exist independently but only within a social and political context. Where the economy is the primary institution of advanced capitalist societies, it must become socialised – that is, socially controlled and organised – if there is to be a future for a post-industrial Left. A corollary of this is the notion that economic decisions are not just the jurisdiction of governments, they require widespread consultation and collective decision-making. It is only through this kind of socialisation of the economy that it becomes more transparent and predictable, and the decisions made concerning it become accountable. On this point it is worth quoting Gorz at greater length:

> The economy is not a machine which operates in a rigorously determinist fashion. It is the outcome of projects, intentions and programmes. The quality of forecasts and adjustments depends on the translation of the intentions and projects into commitments, contracts, collective agreements at branch and enterprise level. This contractualization has many more advantages than disadvantages (as is evident from the Swedish example in particular). By its mere existence, it reduces uncertainty and produces predictability. Plans and commitments made for several years are, in any case, a necessity for the public services and administrative bodies which have to plan their investments and staffing levels several years in advance. The same is true for 'capital-intensive' enterprises. The task of a planning body consists precisely in bringing together and harmonizing sectoral plans, and directing overall general

development towards the priority goals set by government. Forecasting, dialogue, harmonization and orientation have a regulative, stabilizing effect once they are translated into con- tractual commitments.

(Gorz 1994: 113)

In itself, this defence of intervention in the economy to ensure the aims of social justice, democratic decision-making and economic efficiency is not particularly radical. Indeed, even inveterate defenders of relatively free markets such as Hutton (1996, 1997) stress the importance of plan- ning for the long-term health of the economy. But where Hutton stresses long-termism as the basis of economic well-being, Gorz's advocacy of planning is also designed to serve non-economic goals which correspond to post-industrial socialist political principles. In other words, the organ- isation of society and the economy must be conducted in such a way as to provide a conception of social justice that embodies a theory of equality and liberty in which social institutions are designed to 'enable everyone to share equally in the power to control the activities of their own society' (Norman 1987: 155). Thus, in conceptualising liberty, we are not reflect- ing merely on individual liberty as a negative phenomenon, whereby individuals have a nominal ability to act as they please so long as they do not harm others, but rather a theory of human freedom which enables individuals to act positively on their own initiative, combine with others with similar interests *and freedoms* to further common goals and to influ- ence the organisation of society through collective decision-making processes. The key to this conception of liberty is the combination of individuals with others to make collective decisions. This implies that my freedom to make those decisions with others with the same capacities can only take place effectively if they also have the freedom to enter into the combination. In this sense individual liberty to enter into collective agreements is only of value if others have that freedom as well. In other words, individual liberty is meaningful only if it is understood in the con- text of social power which is understood collectively as well as individually.

This is where the concept of equality enters the equation for the post- industrial Left and where it must clearly delineate what rights and obligations will form the basis of a new social contract. Thus the post- industrial Left must outline the means through which it would distribute resources in such a way as to allow individuals to exercise self-determi- nation and also to engage in freely chosen collective activities. In this scenario equality is not conceived as strict equality of income or as a formal equality of opportunity (the rhetoric of which abounds in liberal democracies), but rather as a substantive equality to pursue freely ordained activities. In this sense the desired situation is one where individuals have the freedom to pursue autonomous activities as long as they are also prepared to contribute to the extension of those freedoms to others (which obviously implies some constraints on actions). In terms of individual action this entails being prepared not only to contribute to society but also to help create the conditions under which others are able to contribute as well. This corresponds with our earlier suggestion that individuals should have the right to work and the right not to work at any given period and also that we limit the amount of work for wages we perform at any given time to allow all of those who want to work for wages in the public sphere to do so. In terms of the socialised economy, collective decisions need to be taken and planned about the distribution of work which would demonstrate two key aspects of the politics of the post-industrial Left: the control over the economy that can be exercised by collective participants and the solidarity that can be engendered by such collective decision-making.

However, the implementation of this philosophy – described as a 'moderately radical solution' by one of the few commentators who have engaged with notions of a right to work (Elster 1988: 71-3) – requires a clear framework of rights and responsibilities from which citizens can expect to benefit. The notion of rights related to human needs was evaluated in Chapter 4 and clearly some of these rights would be encapsulated within an unconditional basic income. However, the theory of a citizen's wage suggests that we have a responsibility to ensure the welfare of others and the opportunity for them to work. Clearly, this must involve an outline of the obligations that are reciprocally attached to the rights we enjoy to have certain needs satisfied. This reciprocation of the discourse of rights should provide the basis of a new social contract which would focus both on notions of equality and liberty and the necessity of ecological restructuring (Kallscheuer 1994: 126–7). Moreover, changing the distribution of work is within our control, which makes a right to work more feasible than, for example, the right to a spouse, which is one of the examples Elster uses to refute the right to work (Elster 1988: 74). Where we can argue that both work and love are good for self-esteem in the terms of meeting identity needs, we are in a position to do something positively about the former in terms of socialising the economy while we are not in a position to engineer the conditions under which we guarantee loving relationships for everyone. Equating these two identity needs in a formalistic fashion as Elster does in his *reductio ad absurdum* argument is, ironically, neither logical nor constructive when it comes to practical politics.[8] Elster's argument against the right to work is couched in the terms of productivist discourses which fail to understand that the right, as post-industrial socialists envisage it, would have to take place within the context of the reduction of work for all, the economic right not to work, and the obligation on the part of the state to exercise the power to socialise the economy. As such, the notion of a right to work should be understood as a *distributive* rather than a *redistributive* right (Klausen 1996: 221).

While the literature on rights has been substantial in recent years, notions of obligation and duties have been less documented. Despite his different ideological approach from that articulated here, David Selbourne has argued that the fact that the

> principle of duty is not new, and is much older than the 'politics of rights' which has displaced it in the modern era, does not preclude the claim that it is a path to progress . . . Indeed . . . the performance of duty (to self, fellows, and the civic order) is the morally superior, as well as historically prior, constituent of human association, particularly when it is set against the claims of right.
>
> (Selbourne 1994: 3)

Whereas Selbourne advocates the principle of duty as a key constituent of restoring a rather traditional civic order, obligation takes on a rather different meaning in radical welfare theory as it is designed to create new spaces in which everyone can undertake civic activities free from traditional hierarchical structures. However, discussion of obligations related to welfare need to be carefully formulated as too often they provide a recipe for exclusion and selectivism. Frequently they are used to justify work requirements (or other, often gendered, eligibility criteria) for welfare and workfare schemes which is why so many of the defences of basic income are founded in entitlement to welfare rather than duties of welfare. Gutmann and Thompson argue that a fair scheme which might introduce a work requirement would be centred on 'the principle of basic opportunity [which] includes not only an obligation to work and an obligation to provide conditions that make work acceptable, but also an obligation to respect and enhance the political capacities of citizenship' (Gutmann and Thompson 1996: 306). However, from a post-industrial socialist perspective, this notion of work obligation which permeates contemporary American welfare debates is problematic precisely because it is so firmly work based. It promotes and justifies the ideology of work and, in an economy where there is already insufficient work to go around when it is distributed in line with modern thinking, it provides a means through which those who don't have work become marginalised. In this scenario welfare itself is a negative concept in which the feckless are subsidised and the industrious are penalised. While it may be in the interests of governments enslaved to economic rationality to continue with this distortion of the meaning of welfare, it does little for social cohesion and undermines solidarity between citizens. For the post-industrial Left, welfare is conceived not as a set of social policies but as the *outcome* of policies which promote freedom and equality.

The principle of social obligation remains central to this philosophy but it is not a merely work-based duty that citizens owe, it is the obligation not to submit one's life to the ideology of work and relinquish some of the working hours that are not available to those who don't have a job. In other words, obligation in post-industrial socialist theory is about both participation (in terms of contributing to social wealth) and self-limitation (which entails a duty to contribute to the social welfare of others). This conception of obligation has led Gorz, in line with European Greens, to outline self-limitation as a 'Social Project' (Gorz 1993: 64) precisely because it is not something that can be precisely defined individually but must be subject to collectively defined ideas on sufficiency. For Gorz, sufficiency can only be defined satisfactorily when informed by an 'eco-social politics' which

> aims fundamentally to *restore politically the correlation between less work and less consumption on the one hand, and more autonomy and more existential security on the other, for everyone.* In other words, it involves providing individuals with institutional guarantees that a general reduction in working hours will offer everyone the advantages people formerly sought for themselves: a freer, more relaxed and richer life. Self-limitation is thus shifted from the level of individual choice to the level of a social project.
>
> (Gorz 1993: 65)

Most discussions of obligations with regard to welfare rely on economic notions of the duties we owe in return for social benefits (Gutmann and Thompson 1996), whereas what Gorz is referring to is the definition of rights and obligations in a non-economic fashion. This is the crux of post-industrial socialist theory: the notion that, while markets and spheres of economic rationality are necessary for social reproduction, they must be regulated and placed alongside rather than above other spheres of life which have non-economic interests as their rationale. For Gorz the primacy and domination of economic rationality is the essence of advanced capitalism and the limitation of that rationality provides the impetus for socialism. Just as we can have the 'social' without socialism so we can have capital without capitalism. Thus the roots of post-industrial socialism will be identified 'when economic rationality is assigned a subordinate role in the service of non-economic ends, then society will have emerged from capitalism and founded a different civilization' (Gorz 1993: 66). This approach sets out new parameters for radical welfare debates even if the ideas of the post-industrial Left do not come to fruition.

Whatever the perceived strengths and limitations of the theories outlined here, they provide serious questions for more orthodox viewpoints on the future of social policy and traditional perspectives on the meaning of social welfare.

7

CONCLUSION

The future politics of welfare

In the immediate future mainstream political debates on welfare will continue to be conducted within the rarefied atmosphere created by the economic rationality which characterises advanced capitalism. It seems inevitable that the dominant paradigm constructed within industrial society will constrain the parameters of welfare debates. However, it is clear that the economic developments in advanced capitalist societies cannot provide sufficient resources to generate social welfare because the reference point of work-for-wages is increasingly without solid foundation. In this sense the criticisms launched at modern welfare states identified earlier are likely to become more and more pertinent as the changes in the economy which are now evident set in and render 'workerist' welfare arrangements redundant. Moreover, challenges to models of citizenship which are tinged with the same logic that underpins Western welfare states are also likely to encounter increasing criticism. In short, the models of welfare and citizenship which have provided the backdrop for post-war welfare regimes are likely to face more critical analysis because the very principles which they embody have been undermined. In this sense no amount of tinkering at the edges will be able to resurrect the health of Fordist–Keynesian welfare provision. This suggests that new theoretical proposals need to be created to fill the void left by the redundancy of the 'workerist' model.

Clearly, judging by the fact that guaranteed income models have been largely ignored (especially in the United Kingdom), there has been little attempt to address the exigencies of the contemporary era. Indeed, the absence on the Left of plausible alternatives to Fordist–Keynesian arrangements has left the field free for selectivist and/or neo-liberal approaches to welfare to dominate governmental agendas. The direction of Leftist social policy cannot be surrendered to these hegemonic ideas, as the principles which they embody undermine the ethical values upon which socialism is built, such as universalism and solidarity. However, the opposition to neo-liberal proposals cannot be reiterated and couched within the old welfare discourses of social democratic statism, although some of the principles which they were based upon are still relevant. The latter need to be expressed within a new socio-economic framework, and this has been a major achievement of the representatives of radical Left-libertarianism whether one agrees with their ideas or not. This involves not only the socio-political dimension provided by the radical democratic analysis of post-industrialism but also a genuine engagement with the direction of economic policy-making in the contemporary context. This is a task for the Left generally, not just policy-makers or theoretical commentators. However, the task itself is difficult. It involves a radical reappraisal of what socialism means in the light of the new economy. Moreover, serious and difficult questions need to be addressed with regard to what welfare actually means and how social and economic policies are to interact in ensuring that welfare needs are actually met. Ultimately, it is up to the Left to show why its ideas are more attractive and worthy of support than those which currently dominate the political agenda.

What, then, are the questions which the Left (post-industrial or otherwise) needs to answer? The approach taken here has explicitly highlighted human needs theory as an area in which some potential rests. In itself, this is controversial because universal needs are difficult to identify, but the criteria set out at the end of Chapter 4 show that a theory of human needs does not have to be overly prescriptive by ensuring that they are understood as pluralistically as possible when it comes to need satisfaction. Realistically, though, notions of human needs will always be controversial and open to interpretation, although this does not negate their essential primacy or the political nature of debates over need satisfaction. The point is that the difficulty of defining needs should not deflect us from the task of a needs-based strategy for the redevelopment of welfare strategies. The case advanced here is that the satisfaction of needs will tend to be particularistic in experience and the key to Leftist strategy on welfare is to ensure that individuals have the wherewithal to satisfy their own needs. In this sense it is not a strategy that guarantees that individuals will meet all their needs because they may waste their resources on activities which are not linked to need satisfaction (even if individuals think they are). For this reason a broader welfare strategy will need to provide some services in kind and cannot rely on pure cash transfers as the answer to need satisfaction. Where maximal self-determination is a feasible goal for radical welfare proposals, it is difficult to get away from the necessity of state provision of not only resources to facilitate autonomy (or what Van Parijs calls 'real liberty') but also services which will also further the individual capacity for autonomous action. This identifies a central strategy for future socialist politics of welfare – the primacy of the state in facilitating the conditions under which welfare (both individual and collective) can flourish. Obviously, from the perspective outlined here, this will need to be a self-limiting state which will engender a radicalised and empowered civil society in which individuals can satisfy needs in a particularistic manner.

The theoretical proposal which most clearly corresponds with the ideas outlined above is the notion of a minimum income, although, of course, this could take a variety of forms such as a basic income, a citizen's income, a participation income or a citizen's wage facilitated through a 'second cheque' from the state. These ideas are not really on the policy agenda at the moment (in the United Kingdom at least) but, of course, that should not detract from their primacy and importance. For our purposes they can be divided into proposals which have some kind of work requirement and those which do not. The former are likely to be more difficult to implement than the latter because they entail more than just cash transfers and they impinge on economic policy just as much as social policy. However, it is unlikely that any of these policies could be implemented without greater integration of social and economic policies.

The perception of welfare that is being outlined here is not merely centred on financial circumstances but broader issues of betterment and well-being linked to self-determination. In the contemporary context this points to economic rights linked not only to opportunities to work in the public sphere but also to financial resources when individuals choose to pursue activities which are not rewarded financially. These latter criteria make conditional guaranteed incomes more complicated than pure basic income schemes but they also have the advantage that they avoid the unpopular notion that people would get something for nothing: that is, the freerider objection. None the less, there is nothing to suggest that an unconditional scheme in the shorter term could lead to the more conditional approach identified in the last chapter at a later date and still retain a Leftist dimension. Indeed, *as long as the conditional element applied to everyone* this idea is perfectly suitable for a post-industrial socialist agenda on welfare while choice is provided on an individual basis about the performance of work requirements. However, it is unlikely that a move towards a conditional scheme could be introduced without some acceptance of the principles behind an unconditional scheme, and in this sense the debate between the proponents of different theories remains essential to the furtherance of post-industrial policies (whether socialist or not). But given the lack of attention that these ideas are gaining in mainstream political debates (although their relevance and immediacy is changing this situation in countries such as the Netherlands and Denmark), the central issue to conclude upon is the identification of areas in which these theoretical ideas are going to find currency in future welfare debates.

The step between the immediacy of theoretical ideas and their translation into the policy debates of political practice is a large one, particularly in countries where a willingness to permit governments to intervene positively in economic affairs is rather weak. Obviously, the ideas that have been analysed in this book have implied the readiness of the state to regulate economic policy in such a way that it is placed on an equal footing with, rather than above, social policy. The suggestion is that economic and social policies ultimately should be directed towards similar aims – the security and betterment of individuals and society as a whole. Currently, the economy is regarded as a self-perpetuating entity predicated on the pursuit of growth, profit and accumulation in all capitalist nations, regardless of their degree or form of welfare provision. Thus the economy may be centred on the creation of wealth but rarely is it genuinely concerned with a wholesale redistribution of wealth. Simultaneously, social policy is the poor cousin in the stakes governed by economic rationality. It operates on a lower, *ex post* level, in which welfare is gauged on the premises attached to the logic of the industrial economy. It is only the failure to achieve individual welfare according to the preordained values of the economic system which allows recourse to many forms of state provision. The argument put forward here is that social policy needs to be given a higher priority in the grand scheme of things – it needs to be acknowledged as a key constituent of social reproduction.

However, this is where the main problem arises. There is not necessarily a policy which can reverse the decline of social policy in the current economic climate. In other words the operationalisation of radical social policies can only take place within the context of a broad understanding of the constraints of economic rationality. It is only through the recognition of the constraints which apply in the economy that the underpinning logic of economic relations can change, which is the foundation upon which radical social policies can be built. This necessitates a two-pronged approach centred on both the organisation of the economy and the ways in which social policy can be used in the transformation of society away from domination by the economic sphere. This is not to say that a genuinely *ex ante* position can be created but at least there could be a reasonably clean sheet on which to reconstruct socio-economic relations. The politics of time, that is the construction of a new political agenda based upon radically different patterns of time usage, is not only feasible in the context of the organisation (though not the underpinning logic) of the new economy but it is also philosophically alluring for many – not just the post-industrial Left. Thus, in terms of agency, it holds potential for a coalition of groups and individuals who would benefit from emancipation from the pervasive interference of economic rationality.

At first sight many of these groups may not appear to be immediate candidates for this kind of coalition. For instance, trade unions would appear to be locked into the matrix of the economic system, but on closer inspection the decline in their membership and influence which will be exacerbated in the new economy and the rather selective groups of individuals whom they now represent makes post-industrial socialist politics all the more enticing (Gorz 1989a). A redistribution of work would potentially create a greater constituency for trade union expansion and their power would be enhanced by their role in the widespread economic planning which would need to take place. Moreover, their position as champions of the underprivileged could regain strength as opportunities for alliances with organisations representing those who are currently marginalised from the world of work would increase (Little 1997).

Clearly, there is mileage in the ideas outlined here for Green movements, given the common link of ecological politics. Although the issues raised here may not go far enough for some radical political ecologists, there is obviously some shared ground on issues such as the move beyond the primacy of economic rationality, the view that the logic of the economy must be understood within the context of ecological rationality, and the central political perspective which is embodied within the principle of self-limitation. While not providing solutions for many of the ills identified by political ecologists, the post-industrial Left does offer a form of social organisation in which those problems may be properly addressed. Thus it suggests that an eco-social political space may be opened which could facilitate proper debate over ecological issues that are marginalised within the context of the economic logic which dominates advanced capitalism (Gorz 1993). In this sense even if the post-industrial Left does not provide an ecological blueprint of the good society, it should do more than any other perspective in encouraging dialogue about a post-materialist politics.

A range of other groupings could also enter this alternative coalition. The notion of a redistribution of work and a blend of activities for all could appeal to those opposed to a gendered division of labour. If it embodied opportunities for women and men to achieve an appropriate and more equitable balance between work for wages, domestic work and autonomous activities, then the ideas of the post-industrial Left could help to rectify the situation in which women who are increasingly active in labour markets also continue to perform more work in the domestic arena than men (Tyrrell 1995; Little 1997). Moreover, a redistribution of all work (whether paid or unpaid), accompanied by a guaranteed minimum income for individuals, should also help to facilitate a growth in opportunities for resourced autonomy. This wouldn't solve all of the ills of gender divisions related to work (a comprehensive childcare system might also help, for example) but again it would push them higher up the agenda than is currently the case. However, this issue of the redistribution of work and a new politics of time goes beyond the gender divisions. It also offers sustenance for localised activities in communities, for co-operative projects, and for new strength for institutions in civil society. Thus it can be understood as 'a way in which society explicitly appreciates the real economic significance of activities outside the formal sector' (Loftager 1996: 150). In this sense the redistribution of work and a new politics of time offers considerable potential for radical democrats who want to see a rejuvenation of the public sphere and radical communitarians who advocate the empowerment of associations of interest as intermediary bodies between the state and individuals.

This does not mean that a post-industrial socialist coalition is imminent or that it will necessarily come about. The point is that there is an increasing resonance in Left-libertarian arguments for resourced autonomy, especially in the light of the new economy. This approach when coupled with analysis of the nature of 'post-industrialisation' in the economy provides a unique opportunity for a renewal of socialist politics. The ideas outlined here may not find wholesale support but they do provide an antidote to Leftist politics which are firmly grounded in the discourse and rationality of advanced capitalism. They also highlight theoretical policy options which require analysis and evaluation. When the industrialised economy cannot solve the problems which it creates, as is the case within the new flexibility, then there is increasing pressure on social policy to take up the slack. However, when social policies themselves are also subject to critical pressure due to the nature of the system, then opportunities arise for anti-systemic opposition to be articulated. Whether that opposition is successful or comes to fruition remains to be seen but, in the interim, it is incumbent on the Left to develop theoretical ideas which challenge the dominant order. That, at least, is what is notable about the developing perspective of post-industrial socialism. In short, unlike many other contemporary Leftist perspectives, it encompasses a vibrant critique of the actual *rationality* which acts as the driving force of the economy as well as the philosophical principles which underpin advanced capitalism. For that reason alone it is one of the most resonant critiques of advanced industrial capitalism that there is on offer. At the same time, it is not a prophecy, it requires political will and vision. In Gorz's words:

> [T]here is nothing to guarantee that society will choose the emancipation and autonomy of individuals as its priority or its intended direction, rather than seeking to dominate and exert even greater control over them. What direction the present social changes will take is still an open question; it is today, and will for the foreseeable future remain, the central issue in social conflicts and the key question for social movements.
>
> (Gorz 1989a: 242)

NOTES

INTRODUCTION: THE CONTEXT OF POST-INDUSTRIAL SOCIALISM

1 See Beck (1995: 146-52) for a discussion of the effects on labour of 'risk society'. Similar points are raised by Offe (1996: 36-7)

2 Through the rest of the book I refer to both Left-libertarian and post-industrial socialist ideas. However, the two terms are not synonymous. Whereas post-industrial socialism is usually Left-libertarian in inspiration, the opposite is not always the case. Left-libertarianism may take a variety of forms of which post-industrial socialism is only one. However, the thrust of this book suggests that the latter is the most effective manifestation of the philosophy espoused by the former.

3 As should become clear in Chapter 5, the formula set out by Van Parijs for providing concrete opportunities (the 'leximin') does not correspond with the overall aims of the post-industrial Left.

1 EXPLORING POST-INDUSTRIAL SOCIALISM

1 Other relevant contributions to the origins of the debate over post-industrialism include Touraine (1971) and Kerr et al. (1964). Esping-Andersen (1991: 148-51) distinguishes between 'optimistic' approaches to post-industrialism (which relate to theories such as those of Bell and of Kerr et al.) and 'pessimistic' perspectives which raise the possibility of 'jobless growth' or de-industrialisation. More often than not the latter view has been held by socialist commentators.

2 For a Leftist analysis of post-industrial theorists related to the media, see Lodziak (1986) and Elliot (1982).

3 In this section I have mentioned 'a post-industrial economy', 'the new economy' and 'the current post-industrial economy'. The reason that I have not referred to 'the post-industrial economy' is that there is not one definitive model of what *the* post-industrial economy is. Just as those societies which are deemed post-industrial by commentators such as Esping-Andersen (1993) have very different economies, so we must also recognise that Western economies have moved towards post-industrialism on the basis that transnational corporations have moved operations based on more traditional industrial methods to other parts of the world for a variety of reasons. The focus in this book is on Western capitalist societies and

the potential for post-industrial socialism therein. For an interesting account of the effects of Western post-industrialisation on the Third World, see 'Their Famine, Our Food' in Gorz (1985). For a critical analysis of the notion of a post-industrial economy, see Cohen and Zysman (1987).

4 It is beyond the remit of this book to deal with market socialism in sufficient depth fully to cover all of the issues it raises but Pierson gives the topic extensive coverage and analysis. He also makes the valuable point that there are considerable differences between market socialists on issues such as the role of the state, economic management and ownership (Pierson 1995: 84).

5 This point is addressed in Nove (1983).

6 There is insufficient space here to investigate the totality of Gorz's work but I have attempted to do so elsewhere (Little 1996).

7 The dramatic increase of literature on post-Fordism inevitably means that I cannot do justice to the manifold contributions to the debate here. A recent work which provides a wide coverage is Amin (1994b), which succeeds in giving appropriate space to political and economic geographers and also recognises the degree of opposition to post-Fordism which exists.

8 Ironically, Keith Tester characterises Gorz as a writer who 'has tried to move without bounds' and states that 'the post-modern condition is the intimation of a situation without the boundaries of modernity' (Tester 1993: 51, 31). Tester refers only to Gorz's *Farewell to the Working Class* (written in 1980), which is a critical examination of Marx's theory of the working class as *an historical agent*. As such Tester ignores Gorz's more recent work which is explicitly modernist and looks for the foundations of the future firmly in the present, especially in *Paths to Paradise* and *Critique of Economic Reason*. A similar criticism can be levelled at Pepper, who also has only engaged with *Farewell* (Pepper 1993).

9 The brief treatment of post-modernism in this chapter has been on an explicitly political level. Indeed, it is on this level that post-modernists are most susceptible to criticism. Pepper states that 'Postmodernism tends to place all social conflict in the cultural, not political domain. Its struggle is not to *control* state bureaucracy, but *against* the state' (Pepper 1993: 136). This does not fit comfortably with the explicit role for the state in post-industrial socialism. For a more detailed analysis of post-modernism and the state, see Hoffman (1995).

2 THE POST-INDUSTRIAL SOCIALIST CRITIQUE OF THE WELFARE STATE

1 Useful accounts of the historical development of the welfare state in the United Kingdom can be found in Thane (1982), Deakin (1994), Hill (1993) and Glennerster (1995). A variety of more comparative analyses with other countries in Western Europe (and elsewhere) can be found in Cochrane and Clarke (1993), Deacon (1993), Esping-Andersen (1990), Dixon and Scheurell (1989), Ginsburg (1992) and Lane and Ersson (1994). While the critique of the welfare state developed in this book can broadly be applied to most Western welfare regimes because they are organised along workerist principles, this does not mean, of course, that there is not a variety of welfare states which are organised along very different lines (Pierson 1991: 185–7).

2 It should be noted that despite the influence of Hayek and Friedman on governmental *ideology* in the United Kingdom and the USA, there is much less evidence of them actually influencing *policy* (Mishra 1990: 32–3).

3 While Hayek and Friedman are by far the most well-known neo-liberal thinkers and will be the focus of the analysis here, applications of neo-liberal ideas can also be located in Norman Barry (1992), Seldon (1990) and Willetts (1992).

4 See Chapter 1 for more discussion of markets. Hindess, in an effective analysis of Friedman's polemics, notes that the latter is in favour of 'the market' which, as noted in Chapter 1, is an altogether different concept from 'markets' (Hindess 1987: 122).

5 For more analysis of the role of planning in post-industrial socialism, see Chapter 1.

6 Klein also makes a spurious observation that Gough, O'Connor and Offe should have analysed communist welfare states and the problems therein. While comparative social policy is indeed fundamentally necessary, why these analysts of welfare capitalism should have undertaken this task is unfathomable. Klein is quite right with hindsight to point to the collapse of communist welfare states, but he makes an assumption that they endured the same type of crisis as welfare capitalism. This allows him to accuse 'O'Goffe' of not telling the whole story when, in fact, they were engaging in more limited tasks than he suggests. Might it not be the case that, given the collapse of communist welfare states, there is strong evidence that they were organised in a very different way from welfare capitalism? As Klein is very well aware, others such as Deacon (1983) were conducting comparative research on communist welfare states at that time. For his part, Gough states that 'Klein's attempt at a demolition job is in turn too determinist and all-embracing. There is still a need for a theory of the fiscal limits to social policy in *capitalist* societies' (Gough 1995: 212).

7 The recent work of Ian Gough will be analysed later in this book when I look at the concept of human needs. For more detailed discussion of crisis theory, see Mishra (1984) and Pierson (1991). Gough (1995) provides a useful summary of O'Connor's approach.

8 Dean describes this strand of thought as 'civil society socialism'. He chooses, however, to focus on Offe's earlier neo-Marxist critique of the welfare state (Dean 1995).

9 This section will draw on the elements of feminism and anti-racism which impact most directly on post-industrial socialism. Parts of later chapters will also feed into this debate. However, there is a growing amount of literature in this area which I have insufficient space to discuss. An introduction to feminist perspectives on welfare can be found in George and Wilding (1994). A specifically feminist analysis of social policy is provided by Pascall (1986), Bryson (1992) includes a section on 'Women's Welfare State' and Williams (1989) provides coverage of both the feminist and anti-racist perspectives.

10 The breadth of thought within feminism is reflected in most standard textbooks on political ideologies; see, for example, Eccleshall *et al.* (1994). In terms of social policy and a variety of feminisms, see Williams (1989: 41–86)

11 An interesting example regarding the social construction of gender roles is

165

provided by Baker's examination of foraging societies such as that of the
!Kung San people of Southern Africa (Baker 1987: 118–22).

12 For some interesting statistics from the mid-1980s, see Sherman (1986: ch.
    6). A wealth of useful material linked to this area is contained in Pahl
    (1988).

13 This does not mean that post-industrial socialists have been nearly overt or
    thorough enough about problems related to racial discrimination. Sporadic
    references exist which suggest some commonality of interest with anti-racists
    (Gorz 1994: 3, 17) but the extent of this convergence is undertheorised
    and implicit rather than explicit. My comments here, then, are designed to
    show directions that post-industrial socialism should take as opposed to
    explaining something that already exists. This void in post-industrial social-
    ist literature is part of a broader phenomenon in which anti-racist
    perspectives on social policy have been largely ignored even by feminists who
    share some of the same concerns. More recently Williams (1989), Bryson
    (1992) and Pierson (1991) have helped in signalling this problem and also
    in pointing out that the combined effects of sexism and racism tend to pro-
    duce a very different and harsher experience of the welfare state for black
    women. This produces a more complex relationship with the welfare state
    for black women which is 'something other than the cumulative conse-
    quence of being black and female' (Pierson 1991: 92; see also Wilson 1987).

14 It is beyond the scope of this book to go into detail on specific policies on
    health, education, housing and so on, as our focus is on more general
    theoretical principles which the post-industrial Left believes should under-
    pin policy-making. Therefore, I do not presume to have a recipe for the
    abolition of racism or racial discrimination (Modood 1994). Rather, I will
    attempt in later chapters to outline a universalist way forward which can
    challenge racial disadvantage to some extent.

15 The new economy does not only increase racist problems within nations but
    also between them. See Pierson (1991: 85) for a discussion of migrant
    labour and 'guest workers'.

16 An example of the tendency to overlook Green perspectives related to
    social policy can be found in Jones (1993) which contains virtually nothing
    linked to ecologism despite being entitled *New Perspectives on the Welfare
    State in Europe*. The point is that despite the existence of Green ideas on
    social policy (George and Wilding 1994), they are effectively marginalised
    in debates in the United Kingdom compared with the rest of Europe, where
    they are much more prominent.

17 This is nowhere more clearly highlighted than in the complex and some-
    times contradictory relationship between Greens and the work of André
    Gorz (Kenny and Little 1995; Little 1996: ch. 3).

18 This is a broad and ongoing debate which is not as simple as any dichotomy
    would suggest. For an example of how André Gorz transcends and straddles
    some of these barriers, see Little (1996: ch. 3).

19 Owens argues that Tindale's ideas on sustainability are representative of
    'uncritical rhetoric' which is no substitute for 'rigorous analysis' (Owens
    1994: 209). She believes that Tindale embraces environmental science too
    uncritically in terms of defining limits and points to the reliance of envi-
    ronmental science in framing the nature of sustainable development on
    'politics, economics and ethics' (1994: 213).

3 TOWARDS SOCIALIST CITIZENSHIP

1 An example of the contribution of feminism to new debates on citizenship is the challenge to T. H. Marshall's division of citizenship rights into civil, political and social categories (Bryson 1992). This can obscure important issues which are not easily pigeon-holed such as reproductive rights for women (Held 1989: 201–2). See also Pascall's concern that even the new debate which emerged in the 1980s, let alone Marshall, did not challenge the nature of the relationship between citizenship and dependency (Pascall 1993).

2 For a fuller analysis of Marshall's work than will be covered here, see the recent work of Pinker (1995), Barbalet (1993) and Van Steenbergen (1994).

3 While Marshall was somewhat loose in his idea of the chronological evolutionary development of these rights (Turner 1993a: 7-8), in his defence he did state that these 'periods must, of course, be treated with reasonable elasticity, and there is some evident overlap' (Marshall 1994: 174), particularly with regard to political and social rights. What Marshall meant by 'reasonable elasticity' is debatable, but we should note that elements of social welfare provision developed long before the full franchise was extended to women in 1928 and that the Keynesian welfare state embodied a variety of inequalities between the treatment of men and women which calls into question the application of social rights for the latter. Similar inequalities are highlighted in anti-racist literature on the welfare state (Fraser and Gordon 1994).

4 Marshall did not say too much about economic rights, although his notion that citizenship rights were in an evolutionary process did not preclude the possibility of economic rights becoming more pivotal in the future. Nevertheless, he did suggest that social citizenship embodied the development of full citizenship. The area of economic rights has not received much coverage from most commentators despite the fact that Marshall wrote that 'in the economic field the basic civil right is the right to work' (Marshall 1994: 174). An exception is to be found in the work of Twine, who points out that 'there is in reality no right to sell your labour power in the sense that someone has to buy it' (Twine 1994: 108). In any case we might argue that a genuinely economic right would entail not only the right not to work in a given period but also the right to an income for periods in which one was not working.

5 Civil rights are often assumed when in practice they are frequently undermined by governmental initiatives. In the United Kingdom Twine points to 'an extension of police powers, the interception of communications, restrictions to freedom of assembly, controls on trade union membership, and the "public interest" defence in revealing secret government decisions has been removed' (Twine 1994: 87). From myriad recent examples, one can point to the censorship in the media of representatives of Sinn Fein that occurred in the late 1980s and early 1990s and the ability of the Home Secretary to prevent Northern Irish people from entering Great Britain on an arbitrary basis.

6 A recent example of complacent discussion of the nature of social rights is provided by Rose (1993), who makes a comparative measure of commitment to social rights in European Union countries by the percentage of

GDP which they spend on social policy. On the contrary, social rights cannot be measured by these kind of pecuniary comparisons (interesting and useful though they are). Many Green commentators would also point to the inadequacy of GDP as an indicator of welfare and consequently percentages of it are equally invalid as pointers of commitment to welfare.

7 An exception to this trend can be found in Roche (1992), which covers the notion of social duties in depth.

8 This point will be developed further in Chapter 6, where Gorz's division of society into the macro-social, micro-social and autonomous realms is examined. A comparison of this area with the work of Bill Jordan can be found in Hughes and Little (1996).

9 See Chapter 5 for an analysis of basic income theories which are becoming increasingly prevalent among the West European Left and liberal egalitarians more generally.

4 LEFT-LIBERTARIANISM, AUTONOMY AND HUMAN NEEDS

1 A fuller analysis of these notions of needs is contained in the next section of this chapter. For thorough philosophical discussion of the theory of needs, see Wiggins (1991) and Braybrooke (1987).

2 I have discussed this in relation to the work of Christopher Lasch and the debate over 'the dominant ideology thesis' in Little (1996: 143–7).

3 Cohen notes that we need to be careful not to conflate the meaning of exploitation and oppression as the former refers to the extraction of surplus labour by employers while the latter can take place in a variety of forms, especially of those who are not in employment.

4 Doyal and Gough have produced an extremely rigorous and detailed theory of human need and there is insufficient space here to deal with every facet of their argument. However, I intend to cover in detail those issues which are most relevant to the exposition of a post-industrial socialist position on human needs.

5 See Chapters 2 and 3 for discussions of feminist and anti-racist perspectives on the welfare state and citizenship, and the differences within these ideological groupings.

6 It is a little odd that in the discussion of this approach in the early part of their book Doyal and Gough do not go into any depth about the difference between needs and need satisfaction.

7 Doyal and Gough note Keane's willingness to dispense with a reference to socialism in the part of his book which they focus on here. Having said that, they equate Keane's ideas on relativism with post-structuralism and postmodernism, which is not representative of his work generally and certainly not of post-industrial socialism, to which Keane's ideas have contributed (Gorz 1989a; Bowring 1996).

8 In a footnote Keane correctly rejects Frankel's (1987) contention that these ideas amount to a war of civil society against the state.

9 See Gorz (1994, ch. 9, 'Shorter Hours, Same Pay') for a description of why a limited rate of economic growth is still necessary to carry out socialist social and economic policies as opposed to Green proposals for zero or negative growth.

10 Doyal and Gough believe that a key to critical autonomy is the awareness of other cultures and alternative ways of organising society. For this reason

they ascribe significant importance to cross-cultural education as a means through which critical autonomy can develop (1991: 188). For an analysis of the 'critical' form of autonomy, see Soper (1993: 75–6), who believes that this differentiation of different types of autonomy leaves them open to charges of relativism and ethnocentrism.

11 A full discussion of the strengths and weaknesses of a variety of basic income proposals is contained in the next chapter. Ultimately, none of them quite meets the prerequisites for a post-industrial socialist ideal, but a citizen's wage system might meet those criteria. This idea is discussed in Chapter 6.

5 BASIC INCOME

1 Most advocates of basic income are careful enough to avoid presenting the proposal as a panacea for the problems of the age and argue for it as part of a broader package (Offe 1992), although critics often ignore this fact.

2 Van Parijs's claim that basic income is relatively simple is in contrast to some of the sophisticated philosophical arguments that he and others have presented (Van Parijs 1995). This is so much the case that he has recently pledged himself to a basic income project which is aimed at writing a study that 'could be read by people with all sorts of level of education; a work that would cover the ethics of the proposal, but also the economics, the history, and the politics of it' (Van Parijs 1997b: 21).

3 The proposals of the Commission on Social Justice do not advocate a basic income but do not 'rule out a move towards Citizen's Income' in the future (Commission on Social Justice 1994: 263) if current trends continue. It suggests that the favoured route may be a conditional 'participation income' which fits more closely with some post-industrial socialist proposals (see Chapter 6).

4 Van Parijs does not present basic income as a 'socialist' idea and indeed he believes that some forms of capitalist distribution are more favourable in terms of justice than potentially socialist ones (Van Parijs 1995). Vallentyne (1997: 323) describes him as an egalitarian liberal and Van Parijs himself has discussed the possibility of moving from basic income capitalism directly to communism without a period of socialism in between (van der Veen and Van Parijs 1993a: 155–75). My focus on Van Parijs derives from the theoretical rigour of his work and the large body of work on the topic which he has developed.

5 Van Parijs's theory of justice reflects a climate in political philosophy whereby ideas become depoliticised and overly formalistic (Gray 1995: ch. 1). See Offe (1996: 172–3) for more critical analysis of the growth of rational choice theory (which he regards as anti-sociological) and post-modernism.

6 Norman makes the interesting point that basic income can be located within Walzer's framework of 'complex equality' (Walzer 1983) which holds that if some 'blocked exchanges' are in place, then the distribution of consumer goods becomes irrelevant. Norman, though, adds the caveat that 'large inequalities of income are bound to be also large inequalities of power' and that this is in itself undesirable (Norman 1992: 149).

7 Most basic income theorists argue that there need to be grants on top of basic income for those with special needs, such as the disabled, who may

experience difficulty in reaching a decent standard of living on (what could be a small) basic income. The importance of the issue of standard of living and varying needs is raised by Brian Barry (1992: 133–4).

8 Having said that, Jordan's most recent major contribution to the debate has been criticised by one reviewer for using 'economistic language [which] can be off-putting' (Lister 1997: 82), I would suggest that part of the reason why the basic income debate has been rather stagnant in the United Kingdom is that there is a certain reluctance in social policy to address central issues in economic theory and political philosophy.

9 Like Offe (see note 5), Jordan is scathing of rational choice theory, which he equates with economic individualism insofar as it assumes that individuals focus on 'the critical success of their own lives' (Jordan 1994: 120) rather than locating themselves within social units. This is not to say that Jordan believes individuals are incapable of rational choice, but rather that he believes that choices are made on the basis of other interests as well as self-interest and individual utility maximisation (Jordan 1996: 5–12).

10 This echoes some of the ideas of André Gorz in his *Farewell to the Working Class* in the early 1980s (Gorz 1982). For a full exposition and analysis, see Little (1996: ch. 4), and for an overview of this issue related to welfare, see Kenny and Little (1995).

11 Offe contends that this Left-libertarian perspective is undertheorised, which is one of the reasons for writing this book. For Offe, the Left-libertarian approach to welfare can be identified by an explicit concern with security *and* autonomy.

12 See Clinton *et al.* (1994) and Parker (1989: ch. 10) for analysis of New Right perspectives on negative income tax.

13 I return to these themes in the following chapter.

14 For a full discussion of workfare policies in practice in the USA and a comparison with developments in the United Kingdom, see King (1995).

15 Jordan is much less persuasive when he puts the boot in and equates Gorz's conditional basic income with gulags, concentration camps, Thatcherite training schemes and prison labour (Jordan 1994: 113). He seems to forget that there is a strong vision of autonomous choice in Gorz's theory and a prioritisation of social inclusion which one would assume Jordan might share.

16 My focus here is mainly on the politics and philosophy of basic income and there is insufficient space to deal with the mass of economic theory which has been expounded in this area (Parker 1989; Van Parijs 1992b). However, I do intend to commit a full chapter to the economics of basic income in a book-length study in the future. Other notable treatments and costings of basic income (in the context of Ireland) can be located in O'Toole (1995) and Clarke and Kavanagh (1995).

17 Clinton *et al.* do not highlight the case of children and individual entitlement to basic income. As it would seemingly involve the eradication of child benefits, Jordan (1987: 160) has suggested that there should be a lower rate of basic income for children.

18 It should be noted that Clinton *et al.* are not advocates of a full basic income or radical politics but are, on the contrary, taxation experts from Andersen Consulting.

6 THE CITIZEN'S WAGE AND REDUCED WORKING HOURS

1 I refer to basic income to cover a range of proposals which are based upon unconditional social policies (Purdy 1994). This includes citizen's income schemes, which I prefer to call basic income proposals to differentiate them clearly from the citizen's wage and also because I believe that the conception of citizenship which is involved in them is more limited than that which Gorz proposes in relation to the citizen's wage.

2 See, for example, Gorz (1985) for an early outline of a citizen's wage proposal.

3 Gorz's estimate for the redistribution amounts to a total of 20,000 hours in a lifetime which could be performed in a range of different ways (Gorz 1985; Little 1996: 183). These figures are likely to vary over time and, as such, don't immediately impinge upon the philosophical outline of the citizen's wage which is the focus here. The amount of necessary working hours would be the site of political debate if such a proposal was to be formulated. In his more recent publications Gorz says work requirements for each citizen could average 30 hours per week, or roughly 1,100 in a year (Gorz 1994: 110)

4 A strong proponent of the idea that many activities produce exchange value although this may not be immediately obvious was Friedrich List in 1841 (1991) in the development of his theory of productive powers. However, he did not stress the idea that these activities may have a value in themselves which is non-economic. This point was brought to my attention in discussions with Chris Winch (1997).

5 For Gorz's definition of economically rational work see *Capitalism, Socialism, Ecology* (1994: 53–4). For a broader discussion of economic reason see Gorz (1989a: 138–9) and Little (1996: 101-39).

6 This helps to exemplify why Gorz's proposals should be described as post-industrial socialist rather than Green. Gorz (1994: 103) argues that a reduction in working hours which was not accompanied by growth and higher productivity *would* lead to a decline in income.

7 Bowring provides a strident defence of Gorz on this issue. An example of the commentators he challenges is Schecter, who suggests that Gorz defends a guaranteed minimum income and then notes on the following page that Gorz adds an important caveat to notions of a guaranteed minimum income. In terms of what we have discussed in this book, one cannot defend a guaranteed minimum income and then have caveats about it (Schecter 1994: 161-2).

8 Elster (1988: 72) blithely asserts that work sharing is not an appropriate strategy for combating unemployment without any justification except for the likelihood that trade unions would oppose it. This view is challenged by the interpretations of Gorz (1989a) and Purdy (1988, 1994).

BIBLIOGRAPHY

Amin, A. (1994a) 'Post-Fordism: Models, Fantasies and Phantoms of Transition', in A. Amin (ed.) *Post-Fordism: A Reader*, Oxford: Blackwell.
—— (ed.) (1994b) *Post-Fordism: A Reader*, Oxford: Blackwell.
Andersen, J. G. (1996) 'Marginalization, Citizenship and the Economy: The Capacities of the Universalist Welfare State in Denmark', in E. O. Eriksen and J. Loftager (eds) *The Rationality of the Welfare State*, Oxford: Scandinavian University Press.
Anderson, P. (1994) 'Introduction', in J. G. Anderson and P. Camiller (eds) *Mapping the West European Left*, London: Verso.
Anderson, P. and Camiller, P. (eds) (1994) *Mapping the West European Left*, London: Verso.
Arblaster, A. (1994) *Democracy*, Milton Keynes: Open University Press.
Atkinson, A. (1995) *Public Economics in Action: The Basic Income/Flat Tax Proposal*, Oxford: Clarendon Press.
—— (1996) 'The Case for a Participation Income', *Political Quarterly*, vol. 67, no. 1, January–March.
Avineri, S. and de-Shalit, A. (eds) (1992) *Communitarianism and Individualism*, Oxford: Oxford University Press.
Baker, J. (1987) *Arguing for Equality*, London: Verso.
—— (1992) 'An Egalitarian Case for Basic Income', in P. Van Parijs (ed.) *Arguing for Basic Income: Ethical Foundations for a Radical Reform*, London: Verso.
Bankowski, Z. (1993) 'Social Justice and Equality', in R. Bellamy (ed.) *Theories and Concepts of Politics*, Manchester: Manchester University Press.
Barbalet, J. M. (1988) *Citizenship: Rights, Struggle and Class Inequality*, Milton Keynes: Open University Press.
—— (1993) 'Citizenship, Class Inequality and Resentment', in B. Turner (ed.) *Citizenship and Social Theory*, London: Sage.
Barry, B. (1992) 'Equality Yes, Basic Income No', in P. Van Parijs (ed.) *Arguing for Basic Income: Ethical Foundations for a Radical Reform*, London: Verso.
Barry, N. (1992) *Welfare*, Milton Keynes: Open University Press.
—— (1995) 'Friedman', in V. George and R. Page (eds) *Modern Thinkers on Welfare*, Hemel Hempstead: Harvester Wheatsheaf.

Bauman, Z. (1987) *Legislators and Interpreters*, Cambridge: Polity Press.
—— (1992) *Intimations of Post-Modernity*, London: Routledge.
Bean, P., Ferris, J. and Whynes, D. (eds) (1985) *In Defence of Welfare*, London: Tavistock.
Beck, U. (1992) *Risk Society: Towards a New Modernity*, London: Sage.
—— (1995) *Ecological Politics in an Age of Risk*, Cambridge: Polity Press.
—— (1997) *The Reinvention of Politics: Rethinking Modernity in the Global Social Order*, Cambridge: Polity Press.
Bell, D. (1973) *The Coming of Post-Industrial Society*, New York: Basic Books.
Bellamy, R. (1993a) 'Citizenship and Rights', in R. Bellamy (ed.) *Theories and Concepts of Politics*, Manchester: Manchester University Press.
—— (ed.) (1993b) *Theories and Concepts of Politics*, Manchester: Manchester University Press.
Blossfeld, H.-B., Giannelli, G. and Mayer, K. U. (1993) 'Is There a New Service Proletariat? The Tertiary Sector and Social Inequality in Germany', in G. Esping-Andersen (ed.) *Changing Classes: Stratification and Mobility in Post-industrial Societies*, London: Sage/ISA.
Bowring, F. (1996) 'Misreading Gorz', *New Left Review*, no. 217, May–June.
Braybrooke, D. (1987) *Meeting Needs*, Princeton, NJ: Princeton University Press.
Breitenbach, H., Burden, T. and Coates, D. (1990) *Features of a Viable Socialism*, London: Harvester Wheatsheaf.
Brighouse, H. (1996) 'Transitional and Utopian Market Socialism', in E. O. Wright (ed.) *Equal Shares: Making Market Socialism Work*, London: Verso.
Brown, G. (1994) 'The Politics of Potential: A New Agenda for Labour', in D. Miliband (ed.) *Reinventing the Left*, Cambridge: Polity Press.
Bryson, L. (1992) *Welfare and the State: Who Benefits?*, London: Macmillan.
Burrows, R. and Loader, B. (eds) (1994) *Towards a Post-Fordist Welfare State*, London: Routledge.
Cahill, M. (1995) 'Robertson', in V. George and R. Page (eds) *Modern Thinkers on Welfare*, Hemel Hempstead: Harvester Wheatsheaf.
Calinicos, A. (1989) *Against Postmodernism*, Cambridge: Polity Press.
Carling, A. (1992) 'Just Two Just Taxes', in P. Van Parijs (ed.) *Arguing for Basic Income: Ethical Foundations for a Radical Reform*, London: Verso.
Clarke, C. M. A. and Kavanagh, C. (1995) 'Basic Income and the Irish Worker', in B. Reynolds and S. Healy (eds) *An Adequate Income Guarantee for All*, Dublin: Justice Commission, Conference of Religious of Ireland.
Clarke, J. and Newman, J. (1997) *The Managerial State: Power, Politics and Ideology in the Remaking of Social Welfare*, London: Sage.
Clarke, P. B. (ed.) (1994) *Citizenship*, London: Pluto Press.
—— (1996) *Deep Citizenship*, London: Pluto Press.
Clement, W. and Myles, J. (1994) *Relations of Ruling*, Montreal and Kingston: McGill-Queen's University Press.
Clinton, D., Yates, M. and Kang, D. (1994) *Integrating Taxes and Benefits?*, London: IPPR/Commission on Social Justice Issue Papers, no. 8.
Cochrane, A. and Clarke, J. (eds) (1993) *Comparing Welfare States: Britain in International Context*, London: Sage.

Coenen, H. (1993) 'The Concept of Work in the Trade Unions: Towards a Debate on Economic Rights', in H. Coenen and P. Leisink (eds) *Work and Citizenship in the New Europe*, Aldershot: Edward Elgar.

Coenen, H. and Leisink, P. (eds) (1993) *Work and Citizenship in the New Europe*, Aldershot: Edward Elgar.

Cohen, G. A. (1995) *Self-Ownership, Freedom, and Equality*, Cambridge: Cambridge University Press.

Cohen, S. and Zysman, J. (1987) *Manufacturing Matters: The Myth of the Post-industrial Economy*, New York: Basic Books.

Collinson, H. (ed.) (1996) *Green Guerrillas: Environmental Conflicts and Initiatives in Latin America and the Caribbean*, London: Latin America Bureau.

Commission on Social Justice (1994) *Social Justice: Strategies for National Renewal*, London: Vintage.

Compston, H. (ed.) (1997) *The New Politics of Unemployment: Radical Policy Initiatives in Western Europe*, London: Routledge.

Creedy, J. (1996) 'Comparing Tax and Transfer Systems: Poverty, Inequality and Target Efficiency', *Economica*, no. 63, May.

Currie, E. (1995) 'The End of Work: Public and Private Livelihood in Post-employment Capitalism', in S. Edgell *et al.* (eds) *Debating the Future of the Public Sphere*, Aldershot: Avebury.

Dahrendorf, R. (1994) 'The Changing Quality of Citizenship', in B. Van Steenbergen (ed.) *The Condition of Citizenship*, London: Sage.

Deacon, B. (1983) *Social Policy and Socialism*, London: Pluto Press.

—— (1993) 'Developments in East European Social Policy', in C. Jones (ed.) *New Perspectives on the Welfare State in Europe*, London: Routledge.

Deakin, N. (1994) *The Politics of Welfare: Continuities and Change*, Hemel Hempstead: Harvester Wheatsheaf.

Dean, H. (1995) 'Offe', in V. George and R. Page (eds) *Modern Thinkers on Welfare*, Hemel Hempstead: Harvester Wheatsheaf.

—— (1996) *Welfare, Law and Citizenship*, London: Prentice Hall.

Denney, D. (1995) 'Hall', in V. George and R. Page (eds) *Modern Thinkers on Welfare*, Hemel Hempstead: Harvester Wheatsheaf.

d'Entreves, M. P. (1994) *The Political Philosophy of Hannah Arendt*, London: Routledge.

Devine, P. (1988) *Democracy and Economic Planning*, Cambridge: Polity Press.

Dixon, J. and Scheurell, R. P. (eds) (1989) *Social Welfare in Developed Market Countries*, London: Routledge and Kegan Paul.

Dobson, A. (1990) *Green Political Thought*, London: Routledge.

Dobson, A. and Lucardie, P. (eds) (1993) *The Politics of Nature*, London: Routledge.

Dore, R. (1996) 'A Feasible Jerusalem?', *Political Quarterly*, vol. 67, no. 1, January–March.

Doyal, L. and Gough, I. (1991) *A Theory of Human Need*, London: Macmillan.

Drover, G. and Kerans, P. (1993a) 'New Approaches to Welfare Theory: Foundations', in G. Drover and P. Kerans (eds) *New Approaches to Welfare Theory*, Aldershot: Edward Elgar.

Drover, G. and Kerans, P. (eds) (1993b) *New Approaches to Welfare Theory*, Aldershot: Edward Elgar.

Dunleavy, P. and O'Leary, B. (1987) *Theories of the State*, London: Macmillan.

Eccleshall, R., Geoghegan, V., Jay, R., Kenny, M., Mackenzie, I. and Wilford, R. (eds) (1994) *Political Ideologies*, London: Routledge.

Eckersley, R. (1992) *Environmentalism and Political Theory: Towards an Ecocentric Approach*, London: University College London Press.

Edgell, S., Walklate, S. and Williams, G. (eds) (1995) *Debating the Future of the Public Sphere*, Aldershot: Avebury.

Elliot, L. (1997) 'Enter, the Servants of Change', *Guardian*, 18 January.

Elliot, P. (1982) 'Intellectuals, the "Information Society" and the Disappearance of the Public Sphere', *Media, Culture and Society*, vol. 4, no. 3, July.

Elster, J. (1988) 'Is There (or Should There Be) a Right to Work?', in A. Gutmann (ed.) *Democracy and the Welfare State*, London: Routledge.

Eriksen, E. O. (1996) 'Justification of Needs in the Welfare State', in E. O. Eriksen and J. Loftager (eds) *The Rationality of the Welfare State*, Oxford: Scandinavian University Press.

Eriksen, E.O. and Loftager, J. (eds) (1996) *The Rationality of the Welfare State*, Oxford: Scandinavian University Press.

Esping-Andersen, G. (1990) *The Three Worlds of Welfare Capitalism*, Cambridge: Polity Press.

—— (1991) 'Postindustrial Cleavage Structures: A Comparison of Evolving Patterns of Social Stratification in Germany, Sweden and the United States', in F. F. Piven (ed.) *Labor Parties in Postindustrial Societies*, Cambridge: Polity Press.

—— (1994) 'Equality and Work in the Post-industrial Life-cycle', in D. Miliband (ed.) *Reinventing the Left*, Cambridge: Polity Press.

—— (ed.) (1993) *Changing Classes: Stratification and Mobility in Post-industrial Societies*, London: Sage/ISA.

Farina, F., Hahn, F. and Vannucci, S. (eds) (1996) *Ethics, Rationality, and Economic Behaviour*, Oxford: Clarendon Press.

Ferris, J. (1985) 'Citizenship and the Crisis of the Welfare State', in P. Bean, J. Ferris and D. Whynes (eds) *In Defence of Welfare*, London: Tavistock.

—— (1993) 'Ecological versus Social Rationality: Can There be Green Social Policies?', in A. Dobson and P. Lucardie (eds) *The Politics of Nature*, London: Routledge.

Ferris, J. and Page, R. (eds) (1994) *Social Policy in Transition*, Aldershot: Avebury.

Forbes, I. (ed.) (1986) *Market Socialism: Whose Choice?*, Fabian Tract 516, London: Fabian Society.

Frankel, B. (1987) *The Post-industrial Utopians*, Cambridge: Polity Press.

Fraser, N. and Gordon, L. (1994) 'Civil Citizenship against Social Citizenship? On the Ideology of Contract-versus-Charity', in B. Van Steenbergen (ed.) *The Condition of Citizenship*, London: Sage.

Freeden, M. (1991) *Rights*, Milton Keynes: Open University Press.

Friedman, Marilyn (1992) 'Feminism and Modern Friendship: Dislocating the Community', in S. Avineri and A. de-Shalit (eds) *Communitarianism and Individualism*, Oxford: Oxford University Press.

Friedman, Milton (1982) *Capitalism and Freedom*, Chicago: University of Chicago Press.

Fukuyama, F. (1995) *Trust*, London: Penguin.

Geoghegan, V. (1987) *Utopianism and Marxism*, London: Methuen.

George, V. and Page, R. (1995a) 'Thinking about Welfare in the Modern Era', in V. George and R. Page (eds) *Modern Thinkers on Welfare*, Hemel Hempstead: Harvester Wheatsheaf.

—— (eds) (1995b) *Modern Thinkers on Welfare*, Hemel Hempstead: Harvester Wheatsheaf.

George, V. and Wilding, P. (1994) *Welfare and Ideology*, Hemel Hempstead: Harvester Wheatsheaf.

Gershuny, J. (1993) 'Post-industrial Career Structures in Britain', in G. Esping-Andersen (ed.) *Changing Classes: Stratification and Mobility in Post-industrial Societies*, London: Sage/ISA.

Giddens, A. (1991) *Modernity and Self-identity*, Cambridge: Polity Press.

Ginsburg, N. (1992) *Divisions of Welfare*, London: Sage.

Glennerster, H. (1995) *British Social Policy since 1945*, Oxford: Blackwell.

Glennerster, H. and Midgley, J. (eds) (1991) *The Radical Right in the Welfare State: An International Assessment*, New York and London: Barnes and Noble/Harvester Wheatsheaf.

Goodin, R. E. (1988) *Reasons for Welfare: The Political Theory of the Welfare State*, Princeton, NJ: Princeton University Press.

—— (1992a) *Green Political Theory*, Cambridge: Polity Press.

—— (1992b) 'Towards a Minimally Presumptuous Social Welfare Policy', in P. Van Parijs (ed.) *Arguing for Basic Income: Ethical Foundations for a Radical Reform*, London: Verso.

Gorz, A. (1967) *Strategy for Labor*, Boston: Beacon Press.

—— (1982) *Farewell to the Working Class*, London: Pluto Press.

—— (1985) *Paths to Paradise: On the Liberation from Work*, London: Pluto Press.

—— (1988) 'Making Space for Everyone', *New Statesman and Society*, 25 November.

—— (1989a) *Critique of Economic Reason*, London: Verso.

—— (1989b) 'A Land of Cockayne?', an interview with John Keane, *New Statesman and Society*, 12 May.

—— (1992) 'On the Difference between Society and Community, and Why Basic Income Cannot by Itself Confer Full Membership of Either', in P. Van Parijs (ed.) *Arguing for Basic Income: Ethical Foundations for a Radical Reform*, London: Verso.

—— (1993) 'Political Ecology: Expertocracy versus Self-limitation', in *New Left Review*, no. 202, November–December.

—— (1994) *Capitalism, Socialism, Ecology*, London: Verso.

Gough, I. (1979) *The Political Economy of the Welfare State*, London: Macmillan.

—— (1993) 'Economic Institutions and Human Well-being', in G. Drover and P. Kerans (eds) *New Approaches to Welfare Theory*, Aldershot: Edward Elgar.

—— (1995) 'O'Connor', in V. George and R. Page (eds.) *Modern Thinkers on Welfare*, Hemel Hempstead: Harvester Wheatsheaf.

Gray, J. (1993) *Beyond the New Right*, London: Routledge.

—— (1995) *Enlightenment's Wake*, London: Routledge.

Green Party of Ireland (1989) *Communism and Capitalism – One Down, One to Go: Towards a Sane Economy*, Dublin: Green Party of Ireland.

Gutmann, A. (ed.) (1988) *Democracy and the Welfare State*, London: Routledge.

Gutmann, A. and Thompson, D. (1996) *Democracy and Disagreement*, Cambridge, MA: Belknap Press/Harvard University Press.

Habermas, J. (1976) *Legitimation Crisis*, London: Heinemann.

—— (1987) *The Theory of Communicative Action*, vol. 2, Cambridge: Polity Press.

—— (1990) 'What Does Socialism Mean Today? The Rectifying Revolution and the Need for New Thinking on the Left', *New Left Review*, no. 183, September–October.

—— (1994) 'Citizenship and National Identity', in B. Van Steenbergen (ed.) *The Condition of Citizenship*, London: Sage.

Hahn, F. (1996) 'Some Economical Reflections on Ethics', in F. Farina, F. Hahn and S. Vannucci (eds) *Ethics, Rationality, and Economic Behaviour*, Oxford: Clarendon Press.

Hall, S. (1989) 'The Meaning of New Times', in S. Hall and M. Jacques (eds) *New Times: The Changing Face of Politics in the 1990s*, London: Lawrence and Wishart.

Hall, S. and Jacques, M. (eds) (1989) *New Times: The Changing Face of Politics in the 1990s*, London: Lawrence and Wishart.

Handy, C. (1990) *The Age of Unreason*, London: Arrow.

Harrington, M. (1993) *Socialism: Past and Future*, London: Pluto Press.

Harris, M. (1996) 'Citizenship – New Right and New Labour', *Contemporary Political Studies*, vol. 3, 1885–96.

Hayek, F. A. (1991) *The Road to Serfdom*, London: Routledge.

Healy, S. and Reynolds, B. (1995) 'An Adequate Income Guarantee for All', in B. Reynolds and S. Healy (eds) *An Adequate Income Guarantee for All*, Dublin: Justice Commission, Conference of Religious of Ireland.

Heater, D. (1990) *Citizenship: The Civic Ideal in World History, Politics and Education*, London: Longman.

Held, D. (1989) *Political Theory and the Modern State*, Cambridge: Polity Press.

Hewitt, M. (1996) 'Social Movements and Social Need: Problems with Postmodern Political Theory', in D. Taylor (ed.) *Critical Social Policy*, London: Sage.

Hill, M. (1993) *The Welfare State in Britain: A Political History since 1945*, Aldershot: Edward Elgar.

Hindess, B. (1987) *Freedom, Equality and the Market: Arguments on Social Policy*, London: Tavistock.

—— (1993) 'Citizenship in the Modern West', in B. Turner (ed.) *Citizenship and Social Theory*, London: Sage.

—— (ed.) (1990) *Reactions to the Right*, London: Routledge.

Hirst, P. (1989) 'After Henry', in S. Hall and M. Jacques (eds) *New Times: The Changing Face of Politics in the 1990s*, London: Lawrence and Wishart.

Hirst, P. and Thompson, G. (1996) 'Globalisation: Ten Frequently Asked

Questions and Some Surprising Answers', in *Soundings*, issue 4, Autumn.

Hoffman, J. (1995) *Beyond the State*, Cambridge: Polity Press.

Holmwood, J. (1993) 'Welfare and Citizenship', in R. Bellamy (ed.) *Theories and Concepts of Politics*, Manchester: Manchester University Press.

Hughes, G. and Little, A. (1996) 'Radical Communitarianism in Europe: Social Policy and the Politics of Social Exclusion in the Work of Jordan and Gorz', paper given to the Social Policy Association Conference, Sheffield Hallam University.

Hutton, W. (1994) 'The Social Market in the Global Context', in D. Miliband (ed.) *Reinventing the Left*, Cambridge: Polity Press.

—— (1996) *The State We're In*, London: Vintage.

—— (1997) *The State to Come*, London: Vintage.

Jacobs, J. A. (1993) 'Careers in the US Service Economy', in G. Esping-Andersen (ed.) *Changing Classes: Stratification and Mobility in Post-industrial Societies*, London: Sage/ISA.

Jessop, B. (1994a) 'Post-Fordism and the State', in A. Amin (ed.) *Post-Fordism: A Reader*, Oxford: Blackwell.

—— (1994b) 'The Transition to Post-Fordism and the Schumpeterian Workfare State', in R. Burrows and B. Loader (eds) *Towards a Post-Fordist Welfare State*, London: Routledge.

Jones, C. (ed.) (1993) *New Perspectives on the Welfare State in Europe*, London: Routledge.

Jones, P. (1990) 'Universal Principles and Particular Claims: From Welfare Rights to Welfare States', in A. Ware and R. E. Goodin (eds) *Needs and Welfare*, London: Sage.

—— (1994) *Rights*, London: Macmillan.

Jordan, B. (1985) *The State: Autonomy and Authority*, Oxford: Basil Blackwell.

—— (1987) *Rethinking Welfare*, Oxford: Blackwell.

—— (1989) *The Common Good*, Oxford: Blackwell.

—— (1992) 'Basic Income and the Common Good', in P. Van Parijs (ed.) *Arguing for Basic Income: Ethical Foundations for a Radical Reform*, London: Verso.

—— (1994) 'Efficiency, Justice and the Obligations of Citizenship: The Basic Income Approach', in J. Ferris and R. Page (eds) *Social Policy in Transition*, Aldershot: Avebury.

—— (1996) *A Theory of Poverty and Social Exclusion*, Cambridge: Polity Press.

Kallscheuer, O. (1994) 'Will There Be a European Left? Theoretical and Political Queries', in A. Gorz (1994) *Capitalism, Socialism, Ecology*, London: Verso.

Keane, J. (1988) *Democracy and Civil Society*, London: Verso.

Kellner, D. (1989) *Critical Theory, Marxism and Modernity*, Cambridge: Polity Press.

Kenny, M. (1994) 'Ecologism', in R. Eccleshall *et al.* (eds) *Political Ideologies*, London: Routledge.

Kenny, M. and Little, A. (1995) 'Gorz', in V. George and R. Page (eds) *Modern Thinkers on Welfare*, Hemel Hempstead: Harvester Wheatsheaf.

Kerr, C., Dunlop, J. T., Harbison, F. and Myers, C. (1964) *Industrialism and Industrial Man*, Oxford: Oxford University Press.

King, D. (1995) *Actively Seeking Work: The Politics of Unemployment and Leisure in the United States and Great Britain*, London: University of Chicago Press.

Kitschelt, H. (1995) *The Radical Right in Western Europe*, Michigan: University of Michigan Press, in collaboration with A. J. McGann.

Klausen, J. (1996) 'Citizenship and Social Justice in Open Societies', in E. O. Eriksen and J. Loftager (eds) *The Rationality of the Welfare State*, Oxford: Scandinavian University Press.

Klein, R. (1993) 'O'Goffe's Tale', in C. Jones (ed.) *New Perspectives on the Welfare State in Europe*, London: Routledge.

Kumar, K. (1995) *From Post-industrial to Post-modern Society: New Theories of the Contemporary World*, Oxford: Blackwell.

Kymlicka, W. (1990) *Contemporary Political Philosophy*, Oxford: Oxford University Press.

Laclau, E. and Mouffe, C. (1985) *Hegemony and Socialist Strategy: Towards a Radical Democratic Politics*, London: Verso.

Lane, R. (1991) *The Market Experience*, Cambridge: Cambridge University Press.

Lane, J.-E. and Ersson, S. O. (1994) *Politics and Society in Western Europe*, London: Sage.

Lash, S. and Urry, J. (1987) *The End of Organised Capitalism*, Cambridge: Polity Press.

Leadbetter, C. (1989) 'Thatcherism and Progress', in S. Hall and M. Jacques (eds) *New Times: The Changing Face of Politics in the 1990s*, London: Lawrence and Wishart

Lee, K. (1993) 'To De-industrialize – Is It So Rational?', in A. Dobson and P. Lucardie (eds) *The Politics of Nature*, London: Routledge.

Le Grand, J. and Estrin, S. (eds) (1989) *Market Socialism*, Oxford: Clarendon Press.

Leonard, P. (1997) *Postmodern Welfare: Reconstructing an Emancipatory Project*, London: Sage.

Levine, A. (1996) 'Saving Socialism and/or Abandoning It', in E. O. Wright (ed.) *Equal Shares: Making Market Socialism Work*, London: Verso.

Lindblom, C. E. (1996) 'The Welfare-state Model in Long Historical Perspective', in E. O. Eriksen and J. Loftager (eds) *The Rationality of the Welfare State*, Oxford: Scandinavian University Press.

Lipietz, A. (1993) *Towards a New Economic Order: Postfordism, Ecology and Democracy*, Cambridge: Polity Press.

—— (1994) 'Post-Fordism and Democracy', in A. Amin (ed.) *Post-Fordism: A Reader*, Oxford: Blackwell.

List, F. (1991) *The National System of Political Economy*, New Jersey: Augustus Kelley (first published in 1841).

Lister, R. (1997) 'Poverty and Social Exclusion', *Imprints*, vol. 1, no. 3, March.

Little, A. (1996) *The Political Thought of André Gorz*, London: Routledge.

—— (1997) 'Flexible Working and Socialist Theories of Welfare', *Imprints*, vol. 1, no. 3, March.

Lodziak, C. (1986) *The Power of Television*, London: Pinter.
—— (1995) *Manipulating Needs: Capitalism and Culture*, London: Pluto Press.
Loftager, J. (1996) 'Citizens' Income – a New Welfare-State Strategy?', in E. O. Eriksen and J. Loftager (eds) *The Rationality of the Welfare State*, Oxford: Scandinavian University Press.
Loftager, J. and Madsen, P. K. (1997) 'Denmark', in H. Compston (ed.) *The New Politics of Unemployment: Radical Policy Initiatives in Western Europe*, London: Routledge.
Marcuse, H. (1986) *One-dimensional Man: Studies in the Ideology of Advanced Industrial Society*, London: Ark.
Marquand, D. (1997) 'Blair's Split Personality', *Guardian*, 16 July.
Marshall, T. H. (1994) 'Class and Citizenship', in P. B. Clarke (ed.) *Citizenship*, London: Pluto Press. (taken from *Citizenship and Social Class and Other Essays*, London: Pluto Press, 1991).
Mead, L. (1985) *Beyond Entitlement: The Social Obligations of Citizenship*, New York: Free Press.
Meehan, E. (1993) *Citizenship and the European Community*, London: Sage.
Miliband, D. (ed.) (1994) *Reinventing the Left*, Cambridge: Polity Press.
Miller, D. (1992) 'Community and Citizenship', in S. Avineri and A. de-Shalit (eds) *Communitarianism and Individualism*, Oxford: Oxford University Press.
Miller, D. and Estrin, S. (1986) 'Market Socialism: A Policy for Socialists', in I. Forbes (ed.) *Market Socialism: Whose Choice?*, Fabian Tract 516, London: Fabian Society.
Milner, S. and Mouriaux, R. (1997) 'France', in H. Compston (ed.) *The New Politics of Unemployment: Radical Policy Initiatives in Western Europe*, London: Routledge.
Mishra, R. (1984) *The Welfare State in Crisis*, Hemel Hempstead: Wheatsheaf.
—— (1990) *The Welfare State in Capitalist Society*, Hemel Hempstead: Harvester Wheatsheaf.
Modood, T. (1994) 'Ethnic Difference and Racial Equality: New Challenges for the Left', in D. Miliband (ed.) *Reinventing the Left*, Cambridge: Polity Press.
Moon, J. D. (ed.) (1988) *Responsibility, Rights and Welfare*, London: Westview Press.
Myles, J., Picot, G. and Wannell, T. (1993) 'Does Post-industrialism Matter? The Canadian Experience', in G. Esping-Andersen (ed.) *Changing Classes: Stratification and Mobility in Post-industrial Societies*, London: Sage/ISA.
Nixon, J. and Williamson, V. (1993) 'Returner and Retainer Policies for Women', in C. Jones (ed.) *New Perspectives on the Welfare State in Europe*, London: Routledge.
Norman, R. (1987) *Free and Equal*, Oxford: Oxford University Press.
—— (1992) 'Equality, Needs, and Basic Income', in P. Van Parijs (ed.) *Arguing for Basic Income: Ethical Foundations for a Radical Reform*, London: Verso.
Nove, A. (1983) *The Economics of Feasible Socialism*, London: Allen and Unwin.
O'Connor, J. (1973) *The Fiscal Crisis of the State*, New York: St Martin's Press.
—— (1984) *Accumulation Crisis*, Oxford: Blackwell.

Offe, C. (1984) *Contradictions of the Welfare State*, edited by J. Keane, London: Hutchinson.

—— (1985) *Disorganized Capitalism*, Cambridge: Polity Press.

—— (1992) 'A Non-productivist Design for Social Policies', in P. Van Parijs (ed.) *Arguing for Basic Income: Ethical Foundations for a Radical Reform*, London: Verso.

—— (1996) *Modernity and the State: East, West*, Cambridge: Polity Press.

Offe, C. and Heinze, R. (1992) *Beyond Employment: Time, Work and the Informal Economy*, Cambridge: Polity Press.

Offe, C., Muckenberger, U. and Ostner, I. (1996) 'A Basic Income Guaranteed by the State: A Need of the Moment in Social Policy', in C. Offe (1996) *Modernity and the State: East, West*, Cambridge: Polity Press.

O'Toole, F. (1995) 'The Costings of a Basic Income Scheme', in B. Reynolds and S. Healy (eds) *An Adequate Guarantee for All*, Dublin: Justice Commission, Conference of Religious of Ireland.

Owens, S. (1994) 'Sustainability and Environmental Policy: Five Fundamental Questions', in D. Miliband (ed.) *Reinventing the Left*, Cambridge: Polity Press.

Pahl, R. E. (ed.) (1988) *On Work: Historical, Comparative and Theoretical Approaches*, Oxford: Blackwell.

Parekh, B. (1994) 'Minority Rights, Majority Values', in D. Miliband (ed.) *Reinventing the Left*, Cambridge: Polity Press.

Parker, H. (1989) *Instead of the Dole*, London: Routledge.

—— (ed.) (1993) *Citizen's Income and Women*, London: Citizen's Income.

Pascall, G. (1986) *Social Policy: A Feminist Analysis*, London: Tavistock.

—— (1993) 'Citizenship – A Feminist Analysis', in G. Drover and P. Kerans (eds) *New Approaches to Welfare Theory*, Aldershot: Edward Elgar.

—— (1997) *Social Policy: A Feminist Analysis*, second edition, London: Routledge.

Pepper, D. (1993) *Eco-socialism: From Deep Ecology to Social Justice*, London: Routledge.

Philpott, J. (1997) *Working for Full Employment*, London: Routledge.

Pierson, C. (1991) *Beyond the Welfare State?*, Cambridge: Polity Press.

—— (1995) *Socialism after Communism*, Cambridge: Polity Press.

Pinker, R. (1995) 'Marshall', in V. George and R. Page (eds) *Modern Thinkers on Welfare*, Hemel Hempstead: Harvester Wheatsheaf.

Piven, F. F. (ed.) (1991) *Labor Parties in Postindustrial Societies*, Cambridge: Polity Press.

Pixley, J. (1993) *Citizenship and Employment*, Cambridge: Cambridge University Press.

Plant, R. (1985) 'The Very Idea of a Welfare State', in P. Bean *et al.* (eds) *In Defence of Welfare*, London: Tavistock.

—— (1988) 'Needs, Agency and Welfare Rights', in J. D. Moon (ed.) *Responsibility, Rights and Welfare*, London: Westview Press.

—— (1993) 'Free Lunches Don't Nourish: Reflections on Entitlement and Citizenship', in G. Drover and P. Kerans (eds) *New Approaches to Welfare Theory*, Aldershot: Edward Elgar.

Post, K. (1996) *Regaining Marxism*, London/The Hague: Macmillan/Institute of Social Studies.
Purdy, D. (1988) *Social Power and the Labour Market*, London: Macmillan.
—— (1994) 'Citizenship, Basic Income and the State', *New Left Review*, no. 208, November–December.
Reich, R. (1997) 'New Deal and Fair Deal', *Guardian*, 14 July.
Reynolds, B. and Healy, S. (eds) (1995) *An Adequate Income Guarantee for All*, Dublin: Justice Commission, Conference of Religious of Ireland.
Ritzer, G. (1993) *The McDonaldisation of Society*, Thousand Oaks, CA: Pine Forge Press.
Robertson, J. (1996) 'Towards a New Social Compact: Citizen's Income and Radical Tax Reform', *Political Quarterly*, vol. 16, no. 1, January–March.
Rocard, M. (1994) 'Social Solidarity in a Mixed Economy', in D. Miliband (ed.) *Reinventing the Left*, Cambridge: Polity Press.
Roche, M. (1992) *Rethinking Citizenship: Welfare, Ideology and Change in Modern Society*, Cambridge: Polity Press.
Roemer, J. (1994) *A Future for Socialism*, London: Verso.
Rose, R. (1993) 'Bringing Freedom back in: Rethinking Priorities of the Welfare State', in C. Jones (ed.) *New Perspectives on the Welfare State in Europe*, London: Routledge.
Rothstein, B. (1996) 'The Moral Logic of the Universal Welfare State', in E. O. Eriksen and J. Loftager (eds) *The Rationality of the Welfare State*, Oxford: Scandinavian University Press.
Sabel, C. F. (1994) 'Flexible Specialisation and the Re-emergence of Regional Economies', in A. Amin (ed.) *Post-Fordism: A Reader*, Oxford: Blackwell.
Saunders, P. (1993) 'Citizenship in a Liberal Society', in B. Turner (ed.) *Citizenship and Social Theory*, London: Sage.
Schecter, D. (1994) *Radical Theories: Paths beyond Marxism and Social Democracy*, Manchester: Manchester University Press.
Selbourne, D. (1994) *The Principle of Duty*, London, Sinclair-Stevenson.
Seldon, A. (1990) *Capitalism*, Oxford: Blackwell.
Sherman, B. (1986) *Working at Leisure*, London: Methuen.
Skirbekk, G. (1996) 'The Idea of a Welfare State in a Future Scenario of Great Scarcity', in E. O. Eriksen and J. Loftager (eds) *The Rationality of the Welfare State*, Oxford: Scandinavian University Press.
Smith, J. G. (1997) *Full Employment: A Pledge Betrayed*, London: Macmillan.
Soper, K. (1993) 'The Thick and Thin of Human Needing', in G. Drover and P. Kerans (eds) *New Approaches to Welfare Theory*, Aldershot: Edward Elgar.
Spicker, P. (1993) 'Needs as Claims', *Social Policy and Administration*, vol. 27, no. 1, March.
—— (1993/4) 'Understanding Particularism', *Critical Social Policy*, issue 39, vol. 13, no. 3.
Standing, G. (1992) 'The Need for a New Social Consensus', in P. Van Parijs (ed.) *Arguing for Basic Income: Ethical Foundations for a Radical Reform*, London: Verso.
Steiner, H. (1992) 'Three Just Taxes', in P. Van Parijs (ed.) *Arguing for Basic*

Income: Ethical Foundations for a Radical Reform, London: Verso.

Stoesz, D. and Midgley, J. (1991) 'The Radical Right and the Welfare State', in H. Glennerster and J. Midgley (eds) *The Radical Right in the Welfare State: An International Assessment*, New York and London: Barnes and Noble/Harvester Wheatsheaf.

Taylor, D. (1996a) 'Citizenship and Social Power', in D. Taylor (ed.) *Critical Social Policy*, London: Sage.

—— (ed.) (1996b) *Critical Social Policy*, London: Sage.

Taylor-Gooby, P. (1994) 'Welfare Futures', in J. Ferris and R. Page (eds) *Social Policy in Transition*, Aldershot: Avebury.

Tester, K. (1993) *The Life and Times of Post-modernity*, London: Routledge.

Thane, P. (1982) *Foundations of the Welfare State*, London: Longman.

Therborn, G. (1991) 'Swedish Social Democracy and the Transition from Industrial to Postindustrial Politics', in F. F. Piven (ed.) *Labor Parties in Postindustrial Societies*, Cambridge: Polity Press.

Tindale, S. (1994) 'Sustaining Social Democracy: The Politics of the Environment', in D. Miliband (ed.) *Reinventing the Left*, Cambridge: Polity Press.

Tomlinson, J. (1990) 'Market Socialism', in B. Hindess (ed.) *Reactions to the Right*, London: Routledge.

—— (1995) 'Hayek', in V. George and R. Page (eds) *Modern Thinkers on Welfare*, Hemel Hempstead: Harvester Wheatsheaf.

Touraine, A. (1971) *The Post-industrial Society*, New York: Random House.

Turner, B. (1993a) 'Contemporary Problems in the Theory of Citizenship', in B. Turner (ed.) *Citizenship and Social Theory*, London: Sage.

—— (ed.) (1993b) *Citizenship and Social Theory*, London: Sage.

Twine, F. (1994) *Citizenship and Social Rights: The Interdependence of Self and Society*, London: Sage.

Tyrrell, B. (1995) 'Time in Our Lives: Facts and Analysis on the 90s', *Demos Quarterly*, issue 5.

Vallentyne, P. (1997) 'Self-ownership and Equality: Brute Luck, Gifts, Universal Dominance, and Leximin', *Ethics*, vol. 107, no. 2, January.

van der Veen, R. and Van Parijs, P. (1993a) 'A Capitalist Road to Communism', in P. Van Parijs *Marxism Recycled*, Cambridge: Cambridge University Press.

—— (1993b) 'Universal Grants versus Socialism', in P. Van Parijs *Marxism Recycled*, Cambridge: Cambridge University Press.

Van Parijs, P. (1991) 'Why Surfers Should Be Fed: The Liberal Case for an Unconditional Basic Income', *Philosophy and Public Affairs*, vol. 20.

—— (1992a) 'Competing Justifications of Basic Income', in P. Van Parijs (ed.) *Arguing for Basic Income: Ethical Foundations for a Radical Reform*, London: Verso.

—— (1992b) 'The Second Marriage of Justice and Efficiency', in P. Van Parijs (ed.) *Arguing for Basic Income: Ethical Foundations for a Radical Reform*, London: Verso.

—— (1993) *Marxism Recycled*, Cambridge: Cambridge University Press.

—— (1995) *Real Freedom for All: What (If Anything) Can Justify Capitalism*, Oxford: Oxford University Press.

Van Parijs, P. (1997a) 'Reciprocity and the Justification of an Unconditional Basic Income. Reply to Stuart White', *Political Studies*, vol. 45, no. 2, June.

—— (1997b) 'The Need for Basic Income: An Interview with Philippe Van Parijs', *Imprints*, vol. 1, no. 3, March.

—— (ed.) (1992c) *Arguing for Basic Income: Ethical Foundations for a Radical Reform*, London: Verso.

Van Steenbergen, B. (ed.) (1994) *The Condition of Citizenship*, London: Sage.

Vincent, A. (1992) *Modern Political Ideologies*, Oxford: Blackwell.

Wagner, P. (1994) *A Sociology of Modernity: Liberty and Discipline*, London: Routledge.

Wall, D. (1990) *Getting There: Steps to a Green Society*, London: Green Print.

Walter, T. (1989) *Basic Income: Freedom from Poverty, Freedom to Work*, London: Marion Boyars.

Walzer, M. (1983) *Spheres of Justice*, Oxford: Blackwell.

Ware, A. and Goodin, R. E. (eds) (1990) *Needs and Welfare*, London: Sage.

Weale, A. (1983) *Political Theory and Social Policy*, London: Macmillan.

White, S. (1997) 'Liberal Equality, Exploitation, and the Case for an Unconditional Basic Income', *Political Studies*, vol. 45, no. 2, June.

Wiggins, D. (1991) *Needs, Values, Truth*, second edition, Oxford: Blackwell.

Wilde, L. (1994) *Modern European Socialism*, Aldershot: Dartmouth.

Willetts, D. (1992) *Modern Conservatism*, London: Penguin.

Williams, F. (1989) *Social Policy: A Critical Introduction*, Cambridge: Polity Press.

—— (1994) 'Social Relations, Welfare and the Post-Fordism Debate', in R. Burrows and B. Loader (eds) *Towards a Post-Fordist Welfare State*, London: Routledge.

Williams, K. and Williams, J. (1995) 'Keynes', in V. George and R. Page (eds) *Modern Thinkers on Welfare*, Hemel Hempstead: Harvester Wheatsheaf.

Williams, R. (1983) 'Problems of the Coming Period', *New Left Review*, no. 140, July–August.

Wilson, W. J. (1987) *The Truly Disadvantaged: The Inner City, the Underclass and Public Policy*, London: University of Chicago Press.

Winch, C. (1997) 'Listian Political Economy: Social Capitalism Conceptualised?', unpublished manuscript.

Wright, E. O. (ed.) (1996) *Equal Shares: Making Market Socialism Work*, London: Verso.

INDEX

INDEX

POST-INDUSTRIAL SOCIALISM

  77, 89, 92, 93, 94, 96, 101, 104,
  105, 107, 114, 118, 119, 142,
  148–9, 157
Urry, J. 32
USA 4, 15, 16, 39, 75, 143, 146, 149,
  153
utilitarianism 91
utopia 22, 25, 30, 34, 44, 95

Vallentyne, P. 107, 109–10, 111, 169
van der Veen, R. 169
Van Parijs, P. 1, 10–11, 12, 107,
  108–13, 117, 118, 120, 122, 130,
  142–3, 158, 169
Van Steenbergen, B. 63
Vincent, A. 23

Wagner, P. 35
Wall, D. 55–6
Walter, T. 107

Walzer, M. 92–3, 169
Wannell, T. 21
water 96
Weale, A. 102, 106
welfare state 37–59
White, S. 112–13
Wilde, L. 18
Wilding, P. 47, 53
Williams, F. 36, 47, 48, 49, 52, 166
Williams, J. 38
Williams, K. 38
Williams, R. 88
Williamson, V. 49
Wilson, W. J. 166
work environment 96
workerism 26, 61, 78, 156
workfare 74, 75–8, 137–8, 153
work portfolio 49

Zysman, J. 164

190

Printed in the United States
by Baker & Taylor Publisher Services